T0180743

ETHICS, MEDICAL RESEARCH, AND MEDICINE

ETHICS, MEDICAL RESEARCH, AND MEDICINE

Commercialism versus Environmentalism and Social Justice

Edited by

Andrew Thompson
University of Oregon (retired), Eugene, OR, USA

and

Norman J. Temple
Athabasca University, Athabasca, Alberta, Canada

SPRINGER SCIENCE+BUSINESS MEDIA, LLC

Library of Congress Cataloging-in-Publication Data

Ethics, medical research, and medicine : commercialism versus environmentalism and
social justice / edited by Andrew Thompson, Norman J. Temple.
     p. cm.
   Includes index.
     ISBN 978-0-7923-7103-8   ISBN 978-94-010-0794-8 (eBook)
     DOI 10.1007/978-94-010-0794-8
     1. Medical ethics. 2. Medicine--Research--Moral and ethical aspects. I. Thompson,
Andrew, 1932- II. Temple, Norman J.

   R725.5 .E89 2001
   174'.2--dc21
                                                                    2001038209
ISBN 978-0-7923-7103-8

Printed on acid-free paper

Contents

Contributors

Matthias Egger, MSc, MD
Division of Health Services Research
Department of Social Medicine
University of Bristol
Bristol
UK

Stephen Workman, MD, FRCP(C)
Department of Medicine
Dalhousie University
Halifax
Nova Scotia
Canada

Acknowledgements

I, Andrew Thompson, received encouragement for launching this project from a host of people, too numerous to list. Of the major encouragers, one of them turned out to be the coauthor of the book, Norman Temple; another a coauthor of a chapter, Matthias Egger; and a third a contributing author, Stephen Workman. They are obviously essential to whatever success it enjoys. Two other individuals contributed mightily to the book.

Steven Kaufman, a physician very active and knowledgeable in the antivivisection movement, made voluminous comments on the two chapters on the use of other animals as substitutes for humans. His critique and provision of references were vital to the formation of the two chapters. It took a long time but I think I finally wore him out with my umpteenth revision to the chapters.

John-Arne Skolbekken, associate professor at the Norwegian University of Science and Technology at Trondheim, read and commented extensively on various parts of the book, as well as providing many useful references for enhancing them. He did so in such a complimentary manner that I was always eager to hear from him again.

Many thanks to Susan Stahl for all her help with the final preparation of the manuscript.

Finally, I am grateful to my wife, Marie-Anne, who simply by being there, helps make it all worth while.

Introduction

Andrew Thompson, Norman J. Temple

We humans are an extraordinary species. One of our finest achievements is the development of morality, of a sense of right and wrong. We articulate and then impose this sensitivity upon ourselves in the form of ethical guidelines, rules, regulations, and laws. We have, regrettably, also developed marvelously clever ways of justifying our behavior whenever it runs afoul of these prescriptions. We have, for example, developed the concept of objectivity to guide scientific pursuits and subsequently established rights which undermine the possibility of ever coming close to attaining the goal of being objective -- rights which entitle participating scientists to gain personal, tangible profits from scientific discoveries.

Formerly, we envisaged gods who kept us in place, who reminded us that we were not all-powerful or especially wise. Now we tend to worship our achievements, especially our technological ones, and ourselves. Mary Midgley[1] aptly names this phenomenon, "humanolatry." We have lost our respect for nature in our enthusiasm for changing it to that which suits our shortsighted ends. We must, as she says, "unlearn" this way of thinking. This book is intended to help us in this process. It will take a harsh look at one of our finest achievements, that of medical science, to see how it has gone astray in its enthusiasm for technological "advances." And it will offer a path back to a science that is more in tune with our biosphere, one marked by guidelines which will state what should be obvious, but which have not been stated unequivocally before and consequently not directly confronted. We will start with a short, individual vignette.

Suppose you have a life-threatening heart condition and your physician prescribes a drug, curamax, for it, claiming that taking curamax will significantly improve your chances of survival. Being doubly cursed, you discover through a screening test and subsequent biopsy of tissue that you also have a life-threatening type of cancer. Fortunately, the cancer is thought to be confined to an area of your body that can be completely excised with probably only minor consequences to your subsequent functioning. Now, suppose things are really not as optimistic as your physician has led you to believe. The research which has been done on the heart drug, curamax, indicates it will only extend the life of about three percent of those who take it, and how much their lives will be extended, whether one day or 15 years, is not known. It is true that the likelihood of not dying of the particular disease is greater than three percent, but that doesn't stop you from dying from other things, and the improvement in your overall chances of dying from all causes is only three percent. Nevertheless, you are expected to take curamax for the rest of your days.

Worse still, you find out that the proposed cancer operation has also never been thoroughly researched. There is no sound evidence that you will live a single day longer, even if the cancer is completely removed. In fact, there is evidence to the contrary. The only sure thing is that your quality of life will be diminished due to the consequences of the operation, which could turn out to be major-for you although they are minor for most people. As a result of finding these things out, you feel misled, if not actually lied to, and you are right to feel that way. Something is wrong when products and services are promoted as life saving when the length of the lives extended or their quality is not known with any assurance. Suppose further that this is the norm, not the exception, for modern medical products and procedures. There are still other unhappy consequences, not necessarily directly for you, but for society. These unproven products and procedures cost a lot of money, either because they are extensively prescribed or because, although seldom invoked, the cost per unit is high. As a result, tremendous amounts of societal resources are dedicated to their provision and other societal needs are short-changed to compensate for this misallocation.

Although this example is fictitious, the problem isn't. This will be apparent in the chapters that review some standard treatments for heart disease and cancer. Thus, we have a serious problem. Ignoring the problem and pretending everything that glitters in medical practice is gold will only make for even more misallocation of resources. Since medical research is the fount of many of the products and procedures that constitute the repertoire of medical practice, a logical place to begin a corrective course of action is to set up standards for research which would ensure that the products and procedures that met these standards would be trustworthy. Also required would be that products and procedures resulting from research conducted with the aid of public funding would be affordable to all members of the public who might benefit from them.

What is deemed affordable depends on the world view one assumes. Are remedial treatments of more or less value than preventive measures? Are they of more value than education and other aspects of social justice? Is the health of existing human beings more important than the health and well being of future generations? Are all other forms of life of lesser worth and therefore to be short-changed because of allocation of resources to remedial care for humans? When one lives in a world of finite and largely diminishing resources, such issues become more and more paramount. The answers to these questions will vary according to our overall point of view. Accordingly, we are going to contrast two world points of view in Chapter One, the parochial one which dominates current medical ethics, research, and practice, and a much broader environmental one.

Within the parochial view, what is affordable is quite generous, astonishingly more than for anything else in well-off societies. In fact, the question is not who could afford the resulting product and service but whether sufficient numbers of people and the ruling public officials could be persuaded to purchase it. This is beginning to change, but the cost-effectiveness studies that are done suffer from still another problem, as does the basic research. From the parochial point of view the rights of researchers to profit from their contributions, especially patentable ones, is strongly asserted, and therefore whatever precautions that are taken to curb the influence of these professional and financial interests on the research are mild, in some cases practically non-restrictive. Researchers may also profit from being consultants to the sponsoring commercial firm or having other professional or financial interests in the acceptance and promotion of a product or procedure. Under such conditions, the temptation is to settle for apparent worth of the intervention, rather than proven worth, and the recipients and the public coffer are the losers. Of course, even apparent worth may represent real worth, and over time medical research has done a great deal of good. But to settle for apparent worth when we know we can and should do better would be a mistake.

Accordingly, we will adopt the broader point of view and propose standards which, if met, would go a long way towards ensuring that the research is done in a proper manner and results in interventions which are both affordable and of proven value. We refer to these principles as "Proposed Standards." The standards are ideal, but wholly applicable to fully or partially publicly funded research and could, at least in part, be imposed on the approval process for privately developed products and procedures. Present regulations are either non-existent or far adrift of the Proposed Standards, but they could be made to correspond, given the will to do so. **These are not "Moses down from the mountain" commandments but rather a means of provoking the kind of comprehensive, deep discussion that has been lacking about the deleterious effects of commercialization and professional ambitions on medical research.** Such a discussion would both modify and expand the standards to uncovered areas of research.

The Proposed Standards are intended to protect the general public and do not directly concern those who serve as subjects of medical research. Thus, the purpose of the standards is quite distinct from the international codes and subsequent national guidelines and regulations that have been developed to ensure that people don't become subjects of research without their full, informed consent, or, failing that, the consent of those who can be trusted to look out for their welfare. We refer to the Nuremberg Code, the Declaration of Helsinki, the Belmont Report, the International Ethical Guidelines for Biomedical Research Involving Human Subjects, and such national regulations as the Protection of Human Subjects in the United States Code of Federal Regulations and the Royal College of Physicians, Research Involving Patients Summary of Recommendations.[2,3] This ground has been well covered, though is a "work in progress" given the lack of protection across all nations, especially Third World ones. The Proposed Standards are of a different and much broader genre. They attempt to ensure that the research, itself, is conducted in as objective a fashion as possible, and that it will result in interventions that are not only trustworthy but truly of priority within the broader context of our planetary existence.

INTENDED READERSHIP

The book is intended for both the general educated public and for portions of it. It is directed in particular to politicians and other policy makers; regulators of medical research; biomedical ethicists; editors of medical journals; medical journalists; professors in medical schools and of health-care classes and their students; physicians; environmentalists and advocates of social justice; and, of course, medical researchers. Readers, hopefully, will find that ethics and research are not only of vital importance but can be interesting as well.

PREVIEW OF BOOK

The book is divided into two parts. The first six chapters establish the Proposed Standards and the last five show how they can be applied to various distinct areas of medical research.

Chapter One contrasts two world views and then chooses one as the context for the rest of the book. Chapter Two is dedicated to the determination of Proposed Standards for allowable cost, Chapter Three to biases in research design, and Chapter Four to biases in publication. The Standards that apply to each chapter conclude it.

Chapter Five reviews the scientific case for substituting non-human animals in research intended to benefit humans. It does so in the light of our increased knowledge of differences both within and between species. Chapter Six reviews the moral justification for such research, including the usually unmentioned, but philosophically recognized, one of self-defence. This results in two new Proposed Standards and all of them are then listed.

Chapter Seven applies the standards to the research on statin drugs for heart disease. Chapter Eight applies the standards to the area of medical devices, using the right heart catheter as an example. Chapter Nine does this for screening for cancer of the breast and prostate, and for treatment of cancer of the prostate. Chapter Ten reviews the promises of genetic research, notes its incredible complexity and the need of advanced technology. It questions the hype, the logic, and the ultimate cost of this type of research. The final chapter shows how shifting the priority of medical research from development of increasingly expensive technological interventions to development of effective preventive programs promises not only to be far more beneficial to overall human health but also dovetails with environmental and social justice concerns. The book ends with a postscript overview.

The views expressed in each chapter are those of the authors of that chapter and not necessarily those of all authors.

References

[1] Midgley M (May-June, 1992). Is the biosphere a luxury? *Hastings Center Report*: 7-12.

[2] Vanderpool HY (ed) (1996). *The ethics of research involving human subjects: Facing the 21st century.* (Appendices A through F). Frederick, Maryland: University Publishing Group.

[3] Brody BA (1998). *The ethics of biomedical research: An international perspective.* New York: Oxford University Press.

Chapter One

How Essential is Medical Research?
Andrew Thompson

Nothing exists in a theoretical vacuum, including ethics. Any given ethical perspective is embedded in and a product of a world view. To the degree with which we become aware of our particular world view(s) we will be able to examine and then alter our own ethical perspective. We will start off with two quite different perspectives on the essentialness and importance of medical research. The first is by far the best known, being widely expressed implicitly and explicitly in both the professional and popular media. The second we have seen clearly and forcefully stated only once. We suggest that what is to be promoted ethically, ought not to depend on the basis of better marketing.

We have chosen Thomas Malone[1] to present the first view since the book he co-authored deals with a crucial concern in medical research; that of the danger that medical scientists will lose their objectivity when personal gain or loss is dependent on the outcome of their research (i.e., the problem of conflict of interest). The following quotes are from the opening chapter of the book in which Malone talks about the importance, function, and value of medical research.

> *The economic impact of biomedical research is greatest - though less readily documented -- in the costs and losses that do not occur because illness was prevented, ameliorated, or rapidly cured. Crash fiscal prudence dictates an economic imperative for biomedical research.*
>
> *Medicine and pharmacology should provide solutions to problems associated with aging and for diseases associated with the environment.*
>
> *Effective defences must yet be found for a monotonous catalogue of rampant diseases: cancer, heart disease, many viral infections, AIDS, Alzheimer's and Parkinson's diseases, rheumatoid arthritis and other autoimmune diseases, cystic*

1

A. Thompson and N.J. Temple (eds.), Ethics, Medical Research, and Medicine, 1–8.
© 2001 Kluwer Academic Publishers. Printed in the Netherlands.

*fibrosis, dementia, pain, sickle cell disease, and spinal cord injury,
to name only the most obvious.*

*Despite its economic consequences, the flow of new technology
cannot, in good conscience, be halted or severely impeded, for that
would deprive the public of the new and beneficial procedures that
the biomedical enterprise was intended to develop.*

As you can see, medical research and its attendant technological
developments are considered economically imperative as well as vital to the
future well-being of humankind: common, chronic diseases, genetic
diseases, injuries, pain - essentially an endless list of ailments - "must" be
defended against, and medical solutions "should" be found for even aging
and environmentally-caused illnesses; cost is almost disregarded, since in
one sense the biomedical enterprise is "intended" to do this (i.e., it has a
moral mission). Given this perspective, medical research should have
whatever resources it needs to accomplish its goals, and the pursuit of lesser
goals will have to give way.

Compare this perspective to that of the philosopher Hans Jonas[2]:

*What is it that society can or cannot afford . . . ? It surely can
afford to lose members through death; more than that, it is built on
the balance of death and birth decreed by the order of life. If
cancer, heart disease, and other organic, noncontagious ills,
especially those tending to strike the old more than the young,
continue to exact their toll at the normal rate of incidence
(including the toll of private anguish and misery), society can go
on flourishing in every way.*

*The destination of research is essentially melioristic [that of
improvement]. It does not serve the preservation of the existing
good. . . . Unless the present state is intolerable, the melioristic
goal is in a sense gratuitous, and this not only from the vantage
point of the present. Our descendants have a right to be left an
unplundered planet; they do not have a right to new miracle cures.
We have sinned against them, if by our doing we have destroyed
their inheritance -- which we are doing at full blast: we have not
sinned against them if by the time they come around arthritis has
not been conquered . . . so progress, with all our methodical labor
for it, cannot be budgeted in advance and its fruits received as a
due. Its coming-about at all and its turning out for good (of which
we can never be sure) must be regarded as something akin to
grace.*

Jonas' point of view is dramatically different from that of Malone's. The "musts," "shoulds," and "rights to" are reserved for restoring and preserving the planet for future generations, not for finding cures for present ailments, no matter how deadly or burdensome they are to the individuals who are afflicted by them. Medical progress is "something akin to grace," not a necessity.

A question that should probably be asked of any world perspective is how realistic it is. We will start with that of Malone's. How well do the goals he sets for medical science accord to what is actually possible? If they don't to any significant degree, the titanic amount of resources dedicated to their fulfillment is more akin to pouring money down a drain than to making a judicious investment.

The apparent primary goal is the development of effective defences against or solutions to all major, common ailments, including cancer and all diseases caused by viruses and bacteria. If this is the case, then it is fair to ask what the track record has been in combating these diseases. If it gives little grounds for hope, then the goal and the pursuit of it ought to be abandoned and replaced by something much more modest. We will just look at cancer, but the conclusions would be much the same as if we were to look at tuberculosis, malaria, cholera, and a number of other major diseases.

Lawrent Schwartz[3], a physician and molecular biologist in the Department of Radiation Therapy at Tenon Hospital in Paris and an expert in cancer treatment, recently observed that the incidence and mortality of cancer has increased worldwide since 1981. He notes that: "Progress has been real, but limited mostly to malignancies arising during childhood and early adulthood. For most common tumors, survival rates have increased slightly, but incidence has in many cases soared." He describes cancer cells as "malignant," "malicious," and "clever" and he points out that the use of drugs to treat blood-associated cancers and solid tumors has been stymied by the emergence of resistant cells. His solution? — a shift in research priorities to such things as the lifestyle changes of drinking, smoking, and high-fiber diets -- i.e. to preventive measures.

Bailar and Gornick[4] support this view in their 1997 article. They report that despite the National Cancer Act of 1971 that funded a vigorous cancer research program, there was a six percent increase in age-adjusted mortality from cancer from 1970 to 1994 in the USA. They further comment: "The effect of new treatments for cancer on mortality has been largely disappointing. The promising approach to the control of cancer is a national commitment to prevention, with a concomitant rebalancing of the focus and funding of research."

A more recent article notes: "The percentage of total deaths in the United States attributable to cancer has risen from 16.3 percent in 1965 to 23.3

percent in 1997. . . Even conservative estimates, measuring only the direct costs of treatment, show cost increases from $18.1 billion in 1985 to $27.5 billion in 1990 to $41.4 billion in 1994."[5]

One might reasonably expect just the opposite, given all the billions of dollars expended on the "war on cancer." If one could believe the popular media for the past few decades, there is a promising cure for cancer found almost every week. Careful reading of the articles reveals that the experiments were not on people but on rats or other animals. However, many people assume that what is found to be true of other animals will be applicable to humans also in the near future. This belief also seems unfounded. What is more, Schwartz's characterization of cancer as "clever" applies equally well to the numerous viral and bacterial diseases that have evolved and successfully adapted to the new treatments directed at them.

Smallpox is sometimes used as an example of how modern medicine can successfully eradicate infectious disease. What is not mentioned is that this is the sole success story. It was possible because of a number of factors: there is no nonhuman reservoir; the vaccine is safe and effective even for newborns; and it is long-lasting, inexpensive, and easy to administer.

There are a few other diseases that are theoretically simple to eradicate, such as polio, dracunculiasis (a parasitic disease), and measles. However, the chaotic conditions of our modern world place huge hurdles to such efforts. Overpopulation, mass migration, and political upheaval are some of the destabilizing factors that make it virtually impossible to locate, obtain the permission of, and treat all carriers and potential victims. These factors contribute to pollution-associated plagues as well, such as cholera. Eradication efforts would divert money and staff from basic health services in the poor countries where the diseases are most prevalent with the result that their populations might actually be worse off.[6]

Currently, another direction increasingly dominates medical research and leads to its endless expansion. This is the heavily promoted hope, one can even say "claim," that genetic research will provide the knowledge and means to get the handle on many, if not all, human ailments. Given the importance of this promissory note we shall devote a separate chapter to it. For now, let us content ourselves with the observation that such research is, by and large, tremendously complex, enormously expensive, and of very limited applicability.

This gives rise to another reality check: the question of whom, eventually, would receive whatever treatments would come out of such high-tech research. Certainly the firms, the scientists, and the practitioners involved would profit from the investment but what about the general public? Who, which countries, and which individuals could really afford the interventions that might result?

This question of who would benefit is an ethical issue that concerns all of medical research. A 1999 international forum in Geneva, participated in by about 100 organizations, including the World Health Organization and the World Bank, reported that of the $56 billion expended worldwide in the realm of medical research, less than 10 percent was dedicated to problems that concern 90 percent of the world population. For example, lung infections, diarrhea, and malaria, which are responsible for about 20 percent of all illnesses, received less than one percent of the research money.[7]

Professor Andrew Jameton[8], of the University of Nebraska Medical Center, has urged that the goals of health care and biological research should respond to the worry that a "worldwide public health disaster of major proportions is shaping up." In that connection he notes that "luxury health care as practiced in the U.S. consumes 40 percent of the world's health-care resources on only six percent of the population." This means that Third World countries can expect, at most, a "trickle down" benefit from any new treatment, and then only those that are least expensive. For these countries to spend more on expensive medical treatments would mean less money and resources would be available to direct at readily prevented diseases that are killing them by the millions, diseases spread by polluted water and abetted by poor nutrition.

There is no question that many effective treatments have resulted from medical research, treatments that extend some lives considerably; such as for the treatment of some fatal childhood forms of cancer, and others that ameliorate the lives of many. However, the overall tendency is for research that is devoted to diseases and disorders that plague the aging population of wealthy countries, research which requires expensive, complicated technology. Such high-tech, medical research has a tough case to make if it is to be justified on a practical basis, given its track record with the major killer diseases. It falls even shorter of meeting the ethical norm of just distribution of benefits. These reasons alone are sufficient to make us take Jonas' perspective seriously. Investing in such research would be not a necessity, moral or otherwise, but at most a dispensable "grace."

We will now apply the criteria of realism and of distributive justice to the alternative goal to which Jonas alludes -- "the right [of future generations] to be left an unplundered planet."

In the current political climate, Jonas' goal is also highly unrealistic. The major world powers, who are at the same time the greatest resource users and polluters, have demonstrated time and time again in international conferences their unwillingness to take the steps necessary to stop the deterioration of the Earth's natural resources. However, as it becomes increasingly clear that daily life is being adversely affected by environmental damage, such as sea, air, and water pollution, the chances increase that resources would be diverted to stem and reverse the deterioration. Certainly, it makes more sense to combat the cause rather than to focus our resources on remedial treatments.

Also relevant from an ethical point of view is that the benefits of environmental measures would be more evenly spread. This is especially clear in the case of pollution from greenhouse gases. Pollution of this kind can most easily be stopped by changes in manufacturing and consumption practices in First World countries, and the life forms of the whole planet would benefit from better air and less damage from excess UV radiation that passes through our ozone-denuded atmosphere.

We have adopted Jonas's point of view for this book, as modified by an emphasis on just distribution of available resources. This environmentally and socially conscious perspective will form the background for the ethical standards that are developed in the course of the book. This will be reflected in a number of ways, some direct and some more subtle. The following chapter provides an indirect support for the changes that are proposed. It presents a case for containing the costs of health care to within a proposed limit. **If this proposal were to be adopted, there would be much more money and other resources available to other purposes. Without this limit it will continue to be very difficult for environmentalists and advocates of social justice to find the funds they need to turn things around**.

This, of course, will not happen automatically and they will have to use the reasoning and information provided in the book to argue their case. **They cannot be part of the problem, i.e., unquestionably accept advanced technology medical research as a good and necessary thing – and still fight effectively for their causes**. Nor can they ask that all medical treatments, no matter how expensive or problematic in value, be offered to all that might want them and not to just the well-off and well-insured.

Specific attitudes are especially relevant. One of them is the attitude that most medical researchers have towards other animals, namely that it is appropriate to use them as "cannon fodder" in their "war" on diseases and crippling conditions that affect humans. It is difficult to have this attitude and still wholeheartedly advocate treating other forms of life as worthy of protection and respect. Chapters five and six will challenge the currently dominant view. It arises also in chapter ten on genetic therapy. The research in this area often makes other animals more "human" in order to serve as more appropriate research subjects or for transplantation of their organs into humans.

Sprinkled throughout the chapters will be comparisons between the sums of money expended for single, questionable, but nevertheless standard treatments and the sums available for environmental and social agencies.

As mentioned before, the final chapter will demonstrate how shifting medical research from remedy to prevention can be both less expensive and more effective. One of the important components of prevention is diet. By cutting down our tremendous consumption of animal products, we conserve and even win back our natural surroundings. This is because domestic animals consume much more energy and water, devastate much more land, and pollute much more, than growing crops for a diet consisting primarily of plant food. They thus contribute to an unhealthy environment for all.

Disclaimer

From the proposed perspective many current and currently unquestioned or mildly questioned practices in medical research will be seen as unethical. **By so characterizing them we do not mean to also imply that those who engage in such practices are any more unethical than any other segment of society**. We all have the same motivations for economic security and personal protection, for rewarding work, for health and happiness, and for praise, power, and prestige, and hence the same temptation to minimize broader concerns that might infringe on these pursuits. However, given the position of power of medical researchers in society, it can be argued, as William May[9] has done with regard to physicians, that they have a *noblesse oblige*, a special obligation, to observe the highest ethical standards and not just what is acceptable to their colleagues. It is our hope to inspire at least some of you who are medical researchers, and of those aspiring to such work, to assume this special obligation.

For the rest of you, this book is intended to make you much more aware of the current situation and thus better able to act appropriately, given the opportunity to do so.

References

[1] Malone TE (1992). The moral imperative for biological research. In: Porter RJ, Malone TE, eds. *Biomedical research: collaboration and conflict of interest*. Baltimore: The Johns Hopkins University Press: 3-32.

[2] Jonas H (1989). Philosophical reflections on experimenting with human subjects. In: Beauchamp L, Walters L, eds. *Contemporary issues in bioethics*. Belmont, CA: Wadsworth Publishing Company: 432-40.

[3] Schwartz LH (May 20-21, 1995). The war to cure cancer isn't being won, so emphasize prevention. *International Herald Tribune*: 4.

[4] Bailar JC, Gornick HL (1997). Cancer undefeated. *N Engl J Med* 336:1569-74.

[5] Integrating economic analysis into cancer clinical trials: the National Cancer Institute-American Society of Clinical Oncology Economics Workbook (1998). *J Natl Cancer Inst Monograph* No. 24:1-28.

[6] Stephenson J (1996). A farewell to arms: experts debate global disease eradication efforts. *JAMA* 279: 897-99.

[7] Forschungsgelder ungleich verteilt (March 19, 1999). *Basler Zeitung*: 4.

[8] Jameton AL (1996). Human activity and environmental ethics. In: Thomasas DC, Kusher T, eds. *Birth to death: science and bioethics.* Cambridge, England: Cambridge University Press: 357-67.

[9] May W (1992). The beleaguered rulers: the public obligation of the professional. *Kennedy Institute of Ethics Journal* 2: 25-41.

Chapter Two

Cost, Distributive Justice And *Noblesse Oblige*
Andrew Thompson

Like most people in well-off countries, I had been aware that for a long time government officials have been concerned about the high, ever-expanding costs of health care, but since I was well insured through my university, I had little private concern. A more personal interest in this topic was sparked by a visit to a hospital ethics committee in Eugene, Oregon, arranged by a physician of my acquaintance who was on the committee. My interest was to obtain a personal impression of the kinds of ethical questions that are brought up in such settings and how they are dealt with.

I have no idea how typical the session was but found it interesting that it was apparently run by the chief administrator of the hospital who used it to sound out the committee members on various concerns she had. The major question she posed was, given the hospital's limited budget, should it purchase an expensive piece of equipment. If my memory serves me well, this was a portable kidney dialysis machine. The question prompted a fairly long discourse, and then one of the members boldly and dogmatically stated that he thought that no lifesaving equipment should be denied anyone for reason of cost since lifesaving was the highest of all priorities. This was duly noted by the administrator and shortly thereafter the committee went on to other topics.

I have also read about a mayor who told the new administrator of the local hospital to come to him if he ever needed a lifesaving piece of equipment, that even if it cost a million dollars he would find money for it.

The key word in the above anecdotes is "lifesaving." The other key element is the high-tech equipment. Medicine has succeeded in getting a vice-like grip on the combination of the two elements, which, in our sound bite, image-rich, modern world of communication, is a powerful, persuasive motivator. Even some of the traditional activities associated with lifesaving have been largely usurped by medicine. Take, for example, the popular televised "rescue" series, Baywatch. Although it features the rescue of

9

A. Thompson and N.J. Temple (eds.), Ethics, Medical Research, and Medicine, 9–18.
© 2001 Kluwer Academic Publishers. Printed in the Netherlands.

drowning people, a nonmedical method of lifesaving, it often reaches its dramatic climax with medical rescue teams administering high-tech resuscitation of the apparently lifeless corpse. Life on the edge of death makes for gripping drama and the display of the wonders of modern technology is fascinating. What is actually visible may be only a jagged, bouncing, usually colored wavy line accompanied with pinging sound effects, but the imagination takes over from there and one is suddenly privy to a kind of magic show.

Thus, when funding is required for a medical product or a procedure or a research project, especially if it involves very sophisticated technology and is promoted as being potentially lifesaving -- and what technology cannot -- the knights come to the rescue and somehow the money is found. The degree to which the public has bought into this belief in the magical powers of modern medicine is revealed in a 1994 survey of public attitudes towards health-care systems in three countries: the United States, Canada, and Germany. Thirty-three percent of the Americans, 27 percent of Canadians, and 11 percent of the Germans thought that "modern medicine can cure any illness with access to advanced technology."[1] Many medical scientists, the media who focuses on current or promissory advances of modern medicine, and the commercial firms involved seem hell bent to increase these percentages.

When we have such power of persuasion, we have a corresponding duty to use it with restraint. It would be wrong to capitalize on it for our personal benefit if this is at the expense of society. This is especially true when we know that the persuasive power of the communication exceeds its exactitude.

To start with, the term "lifesaving" is really a misnomer. There is a hint of immortality about it, as if the person whose life is "saved" lives happily ever after, even eternally; one could say that the term is "larger than life." The accurate expression is "life-extending." Using this term leads to further questions, questions that need to be asked if we are going to make wise decisions as to how to react to proposals for medical treatment and research. "How long can we expect lives to be extended?" and, equally important, "What will be the quality of the extended lives?" We will look at the treatment of these questions briefly in this chapter and in more depth in the next one.

When we ask these questions, we recognize that many non-medical activities not only extend lives but enrich them, some of which we will touch on here. However, they consistently lose out to medicine in the competition for available resources because their connection to life extension is more complex and diffuse. Also, what they do and how they do it does not involve glamorous high technology and rarely results in clearly definable, dramatic successes. Rather, they involve prolonged, persistent efforts to change people's behavior or the environment in which they live. That is, by today's standards of recognition, they are a "hard sell." I refer especially to education, social justice, and environmental protection.

Education provides basic knowledge and the tools for acquiring more. It lays the groundwork for suitable employment, which, in turn, provides the means to satisfy basic needs for food, shelter, and personal protection. It also enables people to know enough to make wise choices about their lifestyles. All of these contribute to living longer, healthier, and more satisfying lives.

Social support programs and educational programs respond to both temporary and chronic needs of many kinds. A myriad of special programs strive to provide equal opportunity for all members of a society and enable them to have full and satisfying lives. The most basic programs provide shelter, food, childcare, and educational assistance. Without such aid, many lives would be shortened and not of a quality commensurate with the total resources available in the society.

Another major contributor to extension and quality of life is environmental protection. When we fail to live in a globally sustainable way, we not only eradicate other forms of life, but we also reduce the quality and length of our own lives and that of future generations of all living beings. We do so through the damage, long- and short-term, of pollution, overcrowding, and impoverishment. Because we do not live in a world of irreducible, life-sustaining resources, when we usurp excessive amounts of our common heritage for one purpose, there is that much less for others. Possibly only one resource has increased over the centuries, and that is knowledge. However, its increase is largely in terms of "being on file," since the assimilation of it by any given individual is limited. Hence, we have more and more specialization and less and less knowledge of even other parts of our own fields, much less that of others, and it becomes ever more difficult to achieve broad, comprehensive perspectives.

Another misleading expansion, also a human artifact, is the expansion of national economies. It is this expansion that helps us to ignore the loss of life-sustaining natural resources. In good economic times, in times of budget surpluses, it seems that we are able to do everything that is necessary by giving as much, and maybe a bit more, to environmental protection, as well as to education, social welfare, fighting crime, and the military and yet still continue to expand our health-care expenditures. The journal, *Worldwatch*, reveals this to be an illusion, citing numerous investigations that demonstrate continuing, rapid worldwide deterioration of our environment. We are producing more wealth, primarily for the already well off, at the expense of the basic means for existence of ourselves and future generations. The increased wealth increases consumer spending that, in turn, increases usurpation of our planet's limited resources. We are borrowing from our "principal" and the debt is of staggering dimension.

Health care is the primary culprit for this taking from the future. In the USA the overall expenditure for health care, private and public, is about four times as great as the defence budget, which, in turn, almost equals the combined military spending of all other nations.[2,3] Health care has arrived at this dominant position in a dramatic fashion, expanding its share of the gross domestic product (the total market value of all the goods and services produced by a nation) from 5.2 percent in 1960 to 14.2 percent in 1995, so that it now equals over one trillion dollars.[4] This trend, though less steep, is characteristic of most other First World countries, such as Germany (5.7 percent to 10.5 percent), Switzerland (3.3 to 9.8), Italy (3.6 to 7.7), and Great Britain (4.5 to 6.9). This means that the economic resources available for education, the environment, and all other national priorities have had to give way and do with less, time and time again.

Accordingly, although it may be initially repugnant for some of you to do so, we are going to have to look at the matter of the cost of medical research and the practices it promotes. Medical research is the linchpin factor in the cost of medical practice since it not only is the fount of many of the new products and the equipment that are developed but also of new procedures and practices. And if it is not done well, with the result that products, equipment, and treatments are applied that are of little (or even negative) value, then the cost expands indefinitely for no good purpose.

As pathologists know, one cannot let the emotion of repugnance control one's investigation, and the negative reaction to costing out "lifesaving" research, products, and treatments is no exception. In later chapters we will examine several costly practices that are prevalent and growing in use, for which the supporting scientific evidence is underwhelming. And we will measure this cost against a criterion that we will shortly explain.

But first we need to take care of objections that some readers may have to what we have said about achieving a different, more equitable distribution of resources. We have stated that some of the resources now being expended in ever increasing amounts for medical research and practice should be distributed elsewhere, specifically for education, social justice, and environmental needs. Many will point out that it is naïve to believe that more than perhaps a small portion of the dollars, Euros, and Yens that are not spent for health care will be spent wisely and fairly elsewhere. That is quite true. But there is also no assurance that resources distributed to health care will be spent wisely and fairly and not primarily so as to profit the medical conglomerate rather than the public. And money dedicated to health care is unlikely to be transferred to another budget, regardless of the need.

Thus, to give distributive justice any kind of chance we need to take from the sector which has the most, or rather quit giving so much to it, and distribute it among more appropriate and useful causes.

Another objection might be expressed as: "But isn't reducing health-care costs what Managed Care does, or at least attempts to do? Why do we need another approach and why should we believe any other would work?" First of all, Managed Care and other third party systems are primarily interested in expanding, not reducing, budgets, since they are, by and large, profit-making institutions. They would like to have more public money injected, not less, to take care of the "bad risk" patients: those prone to illness, have chronic illnesses, or are not able to pay. Also, to stay in business they have to offer popular, in-demand services, regardless of their integral value. They can save on services that are not popular to the degree that they are also costly and not truly needed. It is also of benefit to them to offer services that, if successful, will reduce future medical expenses, but their time line is rather short and long-term future benefits are not very interesting. Thus, they are apt to be more sensitive to political pressures and immediate profits or losses than they are to determining and then only offering services of real, rather than apparent, value. The failure to make this distinction between "real" and "apparent" value starts with research, an area over which they have little control, are not primarily concerned with, or expert in.

It is ironic that despite the hue and cry about costs of health care, most of those concerned about it, including medical ethicists, treat it in parochial terms rather than in worldwide or even nationwide terms. That is they worry about the unequal distribution of resources within the health-care sector, and ignore the excessive amount this sector gets. They may even plead for even more resources to be devoted to heath care.

WHEN IS AN INTERVENTION "TOO COSTLY"?

One of the problems with controlling expenditures for medical interventions is that no clear standard exists for determining when a new treatment can be expected to be, or is, too expensive. The vast majority of articles on new treatments avoid this issue, perhaps because they know that if a convincing enough case can be made that it is some kind of miracle cure or the only cure available, even though, perhaps, it doesn't work or doesn't work well for most people, then whatever it costs will be accepted and eventually covered by third party payers.

They also avoid it because they know that it is almost impossible to persuade people that they need to listen to their heads and not their hearts in making decisions as to what is "too expensive" when the intervention is packaged as "lifesaving." We are faced with this challenge in this chapter since we will propose a cut-off point for public funding of research and treatment that is much less than the current, unofficial, soft standard. We don't expect immediate, open-armed acceptance of our "stingy standard"; we only can hope that the reasons for it will be understood and that a germinating process will be engendered that will, in the long run, be persuasive.

This process is abetted by economic analyses of various kinds that are gradually making inroads in well-off countries.[5] No one kind of economic analysis has found universal acceptance and there are disputes as to how best to measure various expenses and exactly what should be included. Some expenses seem to be customarily overlooked, thus providing estimates that are distorted. For example, a review of 97 articles which included cost analysis found that general overhead costs were not included in 91 of them, only 14 mentioned start-up costs, and only 25 considered costs of adverse effects.[6] One plausible explanation for these distorted economic analyses is that many of them were paid for by the company whose product was being evaluated.

UNREALISTIC COST ANALYSES

Often, in doing cost analyses, short-term savings are credited to the experimental treatment and subtracted from its costs. For example, suppose a study finds that fewer of the subjects who take a cholesterol-lowering drug have treatment for heart attacks than those who take a placebo. The costs for the treatment for heart attacks during the period of the study will therefore also be less for the drug-taking group. This difference in costs in favor of the experimental group are then labeled as "savings" and are subtracted from the overall costs of administering the drug. However, these are not really savings, rather they are <u>postponed costs</u>, since all the subjects will eventually die and before they die they will probably suffer and be treated for a number of illness-caused events. There is no assurance that those whose heart attacks were postponed or prevented from occurring will have an overall savings in medical expenses during their lifetimes. In fact, two studies have estimated that eliminating deaths due to many diseases, including heart disease and cancer, would actually <u>increase</u> the cost of health care because these people would live longer and incur more costs for treatment of long-term, chronic illnesses. Only eliminating or reducing these kinds of illnesses, particularly mental disorders and musculoskeletal diseases, would lead to reduction in lifetime health-care costs.[7,8] Therefore we offer the following Proposed Standard.

> **I** In conducting cost analyses of medical interventions, short-term reductions in cost of care that may result from the intervention shall not be counted as "savings" and subtracted from the costs of the intervention, since they are only postponed costs, not real savings. Exceptions could be made for chronic conditions and diseases since they could involve real savings.

MEASURING QUALITY OF LIFE AND SETTING A COST LIMIT

One of the most important variables that should be measured (but rarely is) is postintervention quality of life. The quality of the postintervention life years can be measured in a formula that determines the cost-effectiveness of the intervention. The result is called a "QALY" (Quality-Adjusted Life Year). We will detail this in the next chapter on research design but need to mention it here since it is part of the following proposal.

In view of the lack of any absolute criterion for determining the upper limit of cost we propose a relative criterion. It is based on the average yearly cost of adequately maintaining a minimally sized family in a well-off country; namely, a family that contains one parent and at least one child under 18. By "adequately" we mean enough money to provide adequate shelter, protection, food, education, and basic health care so that each family member will have a good chance of living a satisfying life and making a positive contribution to society. This is a measure of social justice: The total, comprehensive cost of any medical intervention, as measured in terms of the annual cost of the quality life years that are gained (QALYs), should not exceed this limit. That is, we should not extend the lives of some people, most of whom have already lived for many years, at the potential cost of not providing adequate support for others in the society.

There may be a better criterion to offer. This was chosen because it deals with actual costs, not with income, and represents an important, growing, often neglected segment of many societies. We desperately need something like this criterion to have a way of curbing the overwhelming influence that the commercial and medical lobbies exercise.

The default criterion, the one that dominates now, is much higher. It reflects "what the market will bear" and "what can be marketed to the governmental decision makers." It is much more sensitive to the persuasive power of the proponents than to issues of distributive justice.

The proposed new criterion will not prohibit anything, is morally exhortative, and applies only to the distribution of public funding. Wealthy private individuals and private organizations will, of course, make their own rules and personal decisions as to what medical research to support.

II   In determining whether or not public funding should be involved in the research (or treatment) phase of an intervention, the following criterion is proposed: The expense for each extended Quality-Adjusted Life Year (QALY) should be calculated. It should be less than the average yearly expenditures that are required to adequately maintain a minimally-sized family in a well-off country; namely, a family that contains one parent and one child under 18. Research that can be anticipated with reasonable certainty to result in products and procedures that would exceed this amount should not be supported with public funding. The amount includes the cost of the initial intervention and any continuing treatment associated with it throughout the life of the individual.

As an example, in the USA the average amount expended by a single-parent, single-child family unit in 1995 was estimated to be $22,626 (Table 735).[9] This would be approximately $25,000 in 2000. Thus, in the USA no public funding would support research that could be anticipated to result in an intervention that would exceed $25,000 per QALY. The same restriction would apply to already existing interventions. Whether $22,626 was adequate in 1995 to insure a reasonable chance of living a satisfying life and making a positive contribution to the society for each member of the family is not known. If inadequate, and one would suspect as much since it is only $3,236 more than the average amount expended by single persons, this is hardly a reason to increase the ethical allotment to the most well-endowed sector of the economy (Table 734).[9]

Now someone is sure to oppose this standard in a couple of ways, using personally appealing, potentially real situations. For example, what if the ill person was the mother of three young children and without an intervention that would cost, say $25,000 per year, the mother would likely die fairly soon and leave the children without a mother. It would be inhuman to do such a thing and not economic at all, since it would cost a great deal to care for these children and the care may very well not be of the quality that one would expect of a mother.

What is not mentioned is that interventions that cost $25,000 per year of quality life year gained are not typically interventions that make people perfectly healthy. Rather, people who receive such expensive treatments can usually expect to live shortened, partially incapacitated existences. Such people may not be able to meet the "good parent" standard that is implied in the objection. The tragedy that is postponed, losing a parent, can be a tragedy that is extended as well.

To illustrate, suppose an intervention costs $125,000 for initial and continuing treatment and provides the mother an estimated ten additional years of life. If the quality of those extended years is estimated to be, on the average, at 50 percent, then, according to the QALY formula, the cost per extended quality-adjusted year of life would be $25,000. Such a person might be more apt to need care herself than to provide care. But, you may ask, why not five more years of life at full (100 percent) heath? The answer is because in that case such a person would not be estimated to die in five years -- perfectly healthy people generally don't. Much more likely is a losing battle against irreparable damage or an ongoing illness.

On the other hand, suppose this $25,000 per year were to be given to a person with three young children who would otherwise not have the means for equal opportunity for education, healthy nutrition, basic health care, and decent housing in a relatively safe neighborhood. Would not this be a better way of expending such a sum? We simply cannot afford everything, and to continue to give ever more money for purposes of medical research for development of expensive treatments is not a solution; it is an injustice in a "rob Peter to pay Paul" world.

There are others who would present another type of objection, that of needing the special skills of some people. For example, what if a highly trained, and, up to now, very productive 30-year-old secretary were to need an intervention that would cost $25,000 per quality life year gained. Would it not be worth it, simply from an economic point of view? Again, the assumption is that the person would be restored to the same level of health she or he previously enjoyed. This is most likely to be an illusion. It is also likely that someone else could be found and trained, if necessary, that could replace the ill person for a lot less than this amount of money, with the surplus available for other purposes.

It should be mentioned that those who are most likely to require such costly interventions to extend their lives are not apt to be young or fully employed. They are much more likely to be in or near retirement age, and already in poor health.

There will always be exceptions, such as people who fool the experts and do much better than expected as a result of the intervention. On the other hand, there will be those who do much worse. Really appealing cases or cases that appear to justify exceptions on other grounds may well attract private funding. But one should not base a public policy on exceptions and hope.

References

[1] Blendon RJ, Benson J, et al. (Winter, 1995). Who has the best health care system? *Health Affairs*: 221-30.

[2] Organization for Economic Development and Cooperation (OECD) (1999). Table supplied by Suzanne Edam, employee in the Paris headquarters of OECD.

[3] Carrol EE (June 4, 1995). U.S. runs arms race with itself. *Register-Guard*, Eugene, OR: 2C, 4C.

[4] National health care expenditures projections tables (December 12, 1998). *Health Care Financing Administration*. http://www.hcfa.gov/stats/NHE-Proj/tables/default.htm

[5] Strauss MJ, Bleecker GC, Steinwald AB (1993). Cost -effectiveness analyses in a changing health care environment: new issues and challenges. *Eur J Cancer* 29A (Suppl 7): S3-S5.

[6] Balas EA, Kretschmer RAC, et. al. (1998). Interpreting cost analyses of clinical interventions. *JAMA* 279: 54-57.

[7] St. Leger HS (1998). Earlier study of effect on healthcare costs of preventing fatal diseases yielded similar results. *BMJ* 316:1985

[8] Bonneux L, Barendregt JJ, et al. (1998). Preventing fatal diseases increase healthcare costs: cause elimination life table approach. *BMJ* 316: 26-29.

[9] U.S. Bureau of the Census (1998). *Statistical abstract of the United States* (118th edition). Washington, DC.

Chapter Three

Research Design

Andrew Thompson, Norman J. Temple

Research is the fount and caldron of all new medical products and procedures. Thus a distortion of it for purposes that are ill meshed with strictly scientific considerations can have serious consequences. We shall review the aspects of where the research process is most vulnerable to unethical distortions. This chapter is concerned with the design of the research and the next chapter with publication of the results.

Gone are the days, if indeed they ever existed, in which scientific researchers could "do their thing" without interference or pressure. The leisurely, careful pursuit of a notion as to how something might work or investigation of what looks like an undiscovered area may still exist in certain fields, perhaps astronomy where, relatively speaking, it looks as if we do have an eternity to find out more about the universe, but certainly not in any field where a feeling of "urgency" holds sway. Urgency can be created by many things that are not truly vital, but seem so within a particular context or from a certain perspective. Competition, especially when combined with the possibility of gaining or losing money, contributes greatly to a sense of urgency. Neither competition nor urgency are good or bad in themselves but they can contribute to deleterious consequences.

Examples abound of how competition causes urgency: from the desperate attempts of small children to run as fast as they can to catch a ball, evade a pursuer, or hit a homer for their team, to that of spectators at European football matches who beat up and sometimes even kill those who support the other team. Money also causes urgency in many ways and degrees, depending upon whether those seeking and competing for it will have a few more bucks or francs in their pockets to the fear-driven attempts to hold unto their jobs, thinking they may never find another. People even kill themselves in suicidal despair or others in misplaced vindication over what is probably a temporary loss or setback, perhaps even a trivial one, in their finances or financial position. Within a pressure cooker, even a self-created, basically unreal one, people lose perspective.

A. Thompson and N.J. Temple (eds.), Ethics, Medical Research, and Medicine, 19–40.
© 2001 *Kluwer Academic Publishers. Printed in the Netherlands.*

Many fields today are permeated with an oppressive sense of urgency and one of the casualties is ethicality. Loyalty of the employer to the employee and vice versa, clarity and openness of relations, sharing of resources and otherwise supporting one another, and honesty with respect to the worth of one's achievements appear to be becoming rarer virtues. Requests for aid are all too often met with evasion and honest appraisal of one's work is replaced by "hype." Medical research is among the most competitive, money driven enterprises of all and thus extremely vulnerable to such lapses.

We will start our examination with the choosing of the research team. Much of modern research is influenced by parties who have a proprietary interest in what results are obtained, such as pharmaceutical firms who have invested much money in developing new drugs and are thus desirous that studies support their effectiveness. They exercise their influence in a host of subtle, monetary ways, some of which are described below.

PUTTING THE RESEARCHERS ON YOUR PAYROLL

Truly objective, independent research is dependent on having truly objective, independent researchers. Such researchers are an endangered species in the arena of medical research. One reason is that the new frontier of medical science deals with extremely small, delicate "units" and processes that are hard to find, isolate, fix ("mark") their location, and then determine what they do and how they do it. Molecular biology, molecular genetics, microbiology, analytical biochemistry, and other specialties require high-tech equipment and teams of technicians and scientists with a diversity of skills and knowledge. This all means that the price of discovery has increased tremendously.

Such research would obviously be impossible without infusion of considerable amounts of money. Public funding and private, nonprofit, benevolent foundations have not kept up with the demand, and, indeed, are probably less able to do so than ever before. A "gap" has therefore been created. In one sense it is an artificial one since it is not a gap that necessarily "needs" to be fulfilled, especially at any particular pace, but is nevertheless a very real gap to those who wish to be employed in the pertinent areas.

Commercial interests and the scientists that work for them are dependent on new discoveries in order to create new "products" (the definition of which has been expanded, at least in the USA, to include genetically-engineered life forms). These products must be patented to prevent competitors from producing cheaper versions, cheaper since they did not have the expense of developing them. Without new products, the manufacturing companies would lose whatever advantage they have over their competitors when the patents run out. This is in addition to the reduction in sales of some of the products they already control as it becomes evident that these really do not work or that the adverse effects outweigh their benefits. To stay in business, and especially to expand and become more profitable, new products are vital. Such products do not need to be of any real value provided that dispensing physicians and the public believe they are.

Commercial firms are dependent upon governmental and academic scientists for much of the original research that eventually leads to tangible, usable results. They are also dependent on these scientists for independent confirmation of the worth of the resulting product or procedure. Therefore, commercial firms need "outside" scientists. What they have to offer in return is money, the money they make from the public from sales of the new products.

A "marriage" of mutual interests is thus prime for consummation: supposedly independent medical scientists with commercial firms. The one supplies the discoveries and, or, confirms their usefulness, and the other supplies some of the increased funds that are lacking for maintaining a steady rate of new discoveries.

However, as with any marriage, demands and dependencies develop. With monetary relationships, once we become aware that we are beholden to any other party for our perks or livelihood, however indirectly, there is also awareness that we owe something in return, such as a service of equal worth. Even when there seems to be no explicit demand for reciprocation, we tend to be grateful to the "rich uncle" and want to show our gratitude.

All this is very fine and good, except when your work itself is apt to be altered and reduced in value by virtue of the barter. **If what is expected or demanded is not necessarily anything of known, definite, and lasting value, but rather something that can be marketed, then the tendency is to settle for that.** Why? Because it is easier to deliver and if you don't deliver what is wanted you may lose your source of funding and reduce your chances considerably of finding a comparable one.

What actually happens is probably even less apt to arouse soul searching than the above scenario. A norm gets established and people quiet their individual consciences, if indeed they get aroused in the first place, by simply keeping within the norm. After all, if this is what other professionals do, even the most elevated ones, then it must be kosher. Let us briefly look at norms that have been established in three arenas of medical research: academia, governmental agencies, and professional. Each deserves more attention but this is outside the scope of this book.

Academic Research and Industry

Whole universities have formed cooperative arrangements. For example, Monsanto Corporation and Washington University in St. Louis formed a "strategic alliance" in biomedicine as early as July, 1982.[1] Under the agreement, the overall research program is determined by a steering committee chaired by a professor from the university and including five faculty and five representatives of Monsanto. Monsanto supplies the funding for the research projects, including the university's indirect costs. Although officials of both the university and the company claim that there is no undue influence by the company on the selection of research projects for funding, the agreement stipulates that 70 percent of the research be for applied and only 30 percent for basic research. Normally, or at least previous to such arrangements, one would expect the bulk of academic research to be basic rather than applied. The company has the right to review publications or presentations arising from the funded projects and to file any patent applications. It is predictable that the right to review would probably ensure that "industry unfriendly" results could well end up buried in a filing cabinet.

Faculty members can also serve as consultants to Monsanto outside of the formal, contracted arrangements.

FIDA Research foundation, a nonprofit foundation supported by FIDA ApA, an Italian pharmaceutical firm, and Georgetown University entered into an agreement in 1985 to create a joint institute for the neurosciences. A building, the institute's scientific and office equipment, research expenses, and salaries of the employees are all paid for by the FIDA foundation. In return, the university supplies "its good name and the talents of its medical faculty."

University departments that do research in areas that are integral to medical science also may establish arrangements with industry. They may even be dependent upon grants and other arrangements with private industry to continue to survive or to prosper. Also, many of their faculty may have private arrangements with various components of the medical industry, such as being a consultant to a company or an investigator on a company-financed project. And some of these agreements are made under conditions of sworn secrecy with the justification of protecting commercially valuable information.[2]

It is reasonable to assume that these industry-academic partnerships are unlikely to survive unless the contracting industry benefits in terms of patented products and promotion of them through supportive presentations and publications by involved faculty.

Academic researchers have many ways in which to profit from cooperation with industry. They may receive a grant for a research project, with the blessing of the university who usually also gets some financial benefit, such as payment for overhead costs. They may receive an increase in salary paid for by the grant, get their names on any resultant publications, be hired as consultants to the company in some area not directly related to the funded research projects, become stockholders in the company, or they may profit in still other ways. This creates an entire shift in the research orientation from that of simply finding out what is, and why it is so, to developing that which is patentable and thus commercially valuable. It could be argued that the infusion of resources from industry actually does not inhibit basic research but actually enables more basic research to be done in addition to the applied research. However, the entire atmosphere of the academic departments and the research labs is bound to be affected by the new mind-set, with tenure and promotion more apt to be given to those who design projects that lead to financial enrichment of the academic institution.

In a survey of life science researchers of 50 universities who received the most research funding from the National Institute of Health in 1993, 43 percent of the respondents had received a research-related gift in the previous three years independent of a grant or contract, and 32 percent of them reported that the donor wanted prepublication review of articles or reports stemming from the use of the gift. Such gifts included equipment, discretionary funds, and trips to professional meetings.[3]

A Harvard study surveyed 550 companies engaged in biotech research. Twenty percent of their research and development money went to university researchers and 41 percent of the companies reported that at least one trade secret arose out of their university-funded work. Such secrets prevent disclosure of facts that could aid competitors, thus crippling exchange of information of scientific value. Furthermore, "many of the faculty engaged in corporate-sponsored biotech research are also principals in the same companies -- serving on boards of directors, or being paid as consultants. Most of the top-flight researchers enjoy significant equity holdings in the companies." A similar study found that "37 percent of the biotechnology scientists who were members of the prestigious National Academy of Sciences -- a body that advises Congress and the federal government on important matters relating to science policy -- had 'industrial affiliations' casting serious doubt on their objectivity in questions relating to biotech science policies."[4]

There are also informal but nevertheless significant relations, such as the employment of graduate students by the contracting industry and then offering them postgraduate employment later. Regular faculty may spend time in company labs and, in return, company employees may work in university labs as guest workers.

The US federal government sweetened the pie considerably for universities and individual faculty members by a series of legislative acts, beginning with the Bayh-Dole Act of 1980. As a result, inventions by academic scientists on even federally funded research projects were clearly subject to the control of the overseeing institution and were not the property of the government. Universities were also made free to seek industry partnerships and to transfer technical information to the market place. "In effect, the academic medical center had obtained a form of title insurance for its intellectual property, even though this property was generated using federal funds."[1] The usual arrangement is for industry to take out the patents and to pay royalties to the respective department or faculty members.

From the standpoint of two industry executives this is a win-win situation. 'Enlightened self-interest in the public interest' can be defined as pursuing individual goals within a matrix of integrity, ethics, and responsibility. It creates a win-win situation that benefits the public as well as the collaborating parties."[5] The same executives describe regulations designed to protect the public as a major hindrance to academic-industry endeavors.

Universities are aware of the conflict of interest posed by industry-university arrangements and take some steps toward containing their effect. But the rewards for conducting research rigged to maximize the chances of obtaining positive results and for suppressing or downplaying negative results are far greater than the punishments. Short of actually committing provable fraud, no one is going to lose their position or even their reputation. And there is little incentive for undertaking the lengthy, involved process of proving that fraud has been committed.

There was one notable attempt to control this situation in the USA. In 1989 the National Institute of Health proposed conflict of interest guidelines that required those in a position to make decisions about research projects to disclose fully their financial interests and outside professional activities. They also prohibited researchers from holding equity or options in companies.

These proposed guidelines "were widely criticized in the research community because of their restrictions, their prevention of fair remuneration to scientists, and their chilling effect on cooperative ventures between companies and university researchers" [underlining not in original] with the result that they were quickly withdrawn.[6]

A much less restrictive set of rules was developed some years later by the Food and Drug Administration (FDA) that applies to "sponsors of drug,

device, or biologic marketing applications."[7] Drug companies that apply for
licensing of such an entity "have to reveal whether researchers involved in a
drug trial have any commercial interest in the company."[8] But only if the
amount of "commercial interest — stock and patent options, grants, gifts of
equipment, consultation and honorarium fees exceed $25,000! Now this
does not mean that researchers whose investment in the sponsor exceed that
amount would not be allowed to conduct research for it. At most, what
would happen is that the FDA would decide if steps are necessary, "such as
requesting additional independent confirmatory studies or initiating agency
audits, when there is a serious question about the integrity of the data."[7]

**Twenty-five thousand dollars is not a meaningful threshold for
preventing anything. Who would not be inclined to be favorably
disposed toward a sponsor who provided even a quarter of that amount
in gifts and compensation or in whose enterprise one had invested that
much? Actually, there should be zero compensation if truly
independent research is to be conducted. This must include not having
the sponsor pay the basic costs for the research project, the effect of
which is to put all the researchers on its payroll**. We shall formulate a
criterion and propose a remedy for this situation at the end of the chapter.

Should such a criterion be in place and observed, we could anticipate a
major change in the selection of research projects, their designing, and their
publication. As it is now, this whole process is distorted by industry funding
of research. This gives commercial interests subtle and not so subtle control
over the whole research process -- as will be illustrated and documented as
we proceed. The dimensions of this problem are further revealed by a
survey as early as 1988 that reported that "37 percent of the members of the
American Federation for Clinical Research reported that they received
pharmaceutical support for at least part of their research."[9] Other
commercial interests that sponsor research include manufacturers of test kits
and a large variety of sophisticated devices.

The result of such financial contributions can be seen in a review of 107
trials in five leading medical journals. It found that of the 37 trials supported
by the pharmaceutical companies none of them reported that the company's
product was inferior to what was already available in clinical practice and 34
of the 37 reported that the product was better than the traditional treatment.
By contrast, of the 70 trials that were not industry supported, 27 of them
found the traditional treatment to be superior.[10]

A more in-depth study focusing only on 1988-98 articles on cost-
effectiveness of six cancer drugs found that only one out of 20 of the
pharmaceutical company studies reported unfavorable qualitative statements,
for example, that the drug is "not cost-effective." By contrast, nine of 24 of
the nonprofit-sponsored studies reached such unfavorable conclusions.[11]

The fact that more of both groups did not reach a negative conclusion as regards cost-effectiveness may well be due to the implicit standard reported by the study's authors that less than $50,000 per extended life year is generally considered cost-effective. This is twice that of Proposed Standard II.

Another study did a more intensive investigation in that it considered the variety of financial relations of authors to commercial industry. Stelfox and Grace[12] surveyed the 86 listed authors of 70 articles on calcium-channel antagonists with respect to five different types of financial relationships with manufacturers of such drugs or competitive products: support to attend a symposium, honorarium to speak at a symposium, support for an educational program, research funding, and employment or consultation. Sixty-nine authors (80 percent) responded after repeated requests. The majority (63 percent) of the respondents had such a relationship but only two of the 70 articles disclosed this to the readers. All of the supportive authors had one or more financial relationships with at least one pharmaceutical manufacturer, compared to 67 percent of the neutral authors and 43 percent of the critical authors. The differences between the three groups were highly statistically significant.

Recent developments have made the situation even more conducive to the domination of financial interests of all aspects of research and treatment. This is especially evident in relationships with drug companies. An issue of the *New England Journal of Medicine* (May 18, 2000) contained several disquieting articles in this area and an editorial highlights some of their main points.[13] The editor contributes to this discussion by reporting the journal's experience in trying to find a research psychiatrist to write an editorial on the treatment of depression: "We found very few who did not have financial ties to drug companies that make antidepressants." She adds: "The problem is by no means unique to psychiatry. We routinely encounter similar difficulties in finding editorialists in other specialties, particularly those that involve the heavy use of expensive drugs and devices."

The article in this journal by Thomas Bodenheimer[14] describes the systematic change that is taking place in industry-academic relations. New organizations, referred to as "commercially oriented networks of contract research organizations" (CROs) and "site-management organizations" (SMOs), have emerged to facilitate the process of developing sellable products. They are even more permeable to industry influence than academic research centers. These for-profit organizations have been quite successful: "In 1991, 80 percent of industry money for clinical trials went to academic medical centers; by 1998, the figure had dropped precipitously to 40 percent." CROs employ physician-scientists, pharmacists, biostatisticians and managers and may either contract to implement an industry-designed study or design one themselves, usually for the smaller pharmaceutical firms, depending on what is desired. They may then subcontract with SMOs to "organize networks of community physicians, ensure rapid enrollment of patients, and deliver case-report forms to the CRO." The reaction of academia is predictable. In order to regain their lost funding, some universities have already reorganized themselves in similar research networks.

It is not possible to compete in such a market place for commercial funding without compromising independence of investigation in every aspect. Examples abound in this and other articles in the journal. In publication, for example, the report will most likely only be submitted for publication, or submitted in a timely fashion, if it is industry-favorable or can be made to look as if it is. It may well be written by company writers and then circulated, primarily to well known investigators, for their signature. The next chapter will go into this in much more depth.

GOVERNMENT RELATIONS WITH INDUSTRY

The Bayh-Dole Act and the Stevenson-Wyder Technology Innovation Act, both of 1980, were the forerunners of the US federal government's cooperation with industry in producing commercially sold "technological innovations." The Stevenson-Wyder Act required that each agency with federal laboratories allocate at least one-half of a percent of its research and development budget to support technological transfer. First preference for this transference from federal labs to nongovernmental entities was initially given to nonprofit organizations and small business firms but a presidential directive in 1983 made such transfers equally available to large businesses as well.[15]

Also, beginning in August, 1980, federal scientists were able to get approval for doing "outside work" for industry, such as giving lectures for an honorarium. One rationale for this change was to compensate for the generally lower salaries of National Institute of Health (NIH) scientists compared to scientists in academia. The regulations were broadened in 1985: NIH scientists were "permitted to consult, on their own time, for profit-making companies so long as no government information not already in the public domain (that is, published or presented at an open meeting) was given to the company as a result of the paid consultation." They could earn as much as $25,000 annually from such consultations, "subject to a variety of restrictions and safeguards." However, they were not allowed to hold stock or stock options in the company.

The Federal Technology Transfer Act of 1986 further stimulated the commercialization of research from federal labs by allowing commercial firms to have the exclusive license for resulting technological innovations. In return, the government inventor and the lab involved receive part of the royalties. It also authorized the government to contribute resources, such as personnel, equipment, and material to a commercial collaborator, but not funds, and to receive similar resources, including funds, from such collaborators.

Thus a "win-win" situation, similar to that between academia and industry, is created in which government and industry both profit from research devoted to the development of marketable products. Federal labs may also be affected in similar ways. It is to be doubted, although vehemently denied by those concerned, that the public interest comes first in such arrangements. True, the public is the intended recipient of these technological innovations, but unless the research findings are truly needed and trustworthy, the public does not benefit. On the contrary it foots the bills and enriches those who develop these innovations, and, in the process diverts resources from more urgent and important pursuits.

Other countries have different regulations respecting conflict of interest but the USA both dominates much of the research scene and is the largest single market for such products.[16] Thus it has a powerful influence on the standards set in the rest of the world.

PROFESSIONAL MEDICINE'S RELATIONSHIP WITH INDUSTRY

The American Medical Association addressed the issue of conflict of interest in medical center/industry research relationships in 1990.[17] It recognized the risks inherent in such relationships: bias, less time for patient care or other clinical responsibilities, more costs to patients, and less willingness to share "profitable" knowledge. However, the general tone of the report was supportive of such relationships. "The transformation of technology from basic into clinical laboratories and finally into useful products with commercial value is an accepted and laudable practice that provides a sound basis for social, economic, and scientific policy." It mitigates this statement by the following: "Full disclosure, however, is an essential ingredient to the success of this venture."

We concur with this latter part and point out, as it does: "Disclosure is, to be sure, necessary, but discourse does not mitigate the risks — it only announces that the risk is present." Recognizing that further ethical guidelines are required, it states that such guidelines "ultimately turn on two principles. First, the researcher may ethically share in the economic rewards of his or her efforts." The second guideline is stated somewhat obliquely: "The principle that the researcher may benefit from his or her efforts is limited by the proviso that potential sources of bias in research should always be minimized. . ." The specific example given is that once an investigator becomes involved, or potentially involved in a project for a company, the investigator should not buy or sell the company's stock until the involvement ends and the results are made public. However, they can have other economic ties, such as serving as consultants for the company, as long as they are not overpaid for their efforts.

This claim that investigators are "ethically" entitled to a share of any profits made from their work is a questionable one. If accepted, the door is wide open for bias to enter, and, in fact, there is no real prevention against it. Thus the harm that can result from such a policy is far more extensive than the benefit, which consists only of more profit for those already well paid. Researchers are certainly entitled to a salary for their work and scientific recognition for their work, but financial profit from their discoveries? How would it be if psychotherapists would join the act and demand their fair share of any increased profits that their clients enjoy, presumably because of the therapist's efforts? Or teachers of their pupils' earnings? Or police officers from recovering stolen property. Or government officials who sign trade agreements? Where is the line to be drawn between doing one's job and making bonus profits from so doing it? And if we were to allow therapists, teachers, police, and officials to share in profits, would it not alter their objectivity and distort their sense of benevolence towards those dependent on them?

The expression, "acceptable and laudable practice," warrants special attention. Acceptable practices are not necessarily ethical ones. For example, it may be acceptable to bribe public officials in many cultures but this does not make it ethical, and certainly not laudable. What ought to be accepted is the question that is relevant from an ethical point of view. To call something "laudable" is not argument: it is attempting to convince without any added substance. The sharing of profits by investigators acts to the detriment of the public insofar as it inevitably biases the scientists to develop products that are commercially interesting but may be of little or even negative value to the public. And when the investigators are also in charge of the care of the patients, the focus on potentially rewarding experimentation diminishes their attention to their patients' well being.

It is abundantly clear that the norms in industry, academia, the federal government, and in the medical profession in the USA are wide open to substantial conflicts of interests between individual profit and public interest. Let us see in more detail how this can affect the research that is done. This discussion is primarily relevant to the stage of research that should be conducted prior to approval on new products and procedures: clinical trials.

RIGGING THE STUDY

There is no great difficulty in designing a study so that the results will be industry-friendly. For example, suppose you have a vested interest in showing that a new cholesterol-lowering drug is effective in preventing heart disease. You know that aspirin is generally recognized as being fairly effective in such prevention, and will probably have less deleterious side effects than this new drug. It is also many, many times less expensive. You are also aware that numerous studies have indicated that diets greatly reduced in saturated fat are strikingly successful in prevention and amelioration of heart disease, much more so than the current medical standard of holding total fat content to under 30 percent of energy intake.

If your purpose is to find out whether this drug truly adds anything of value to what is already available in standard treatment, you would prescribe aspirin and perhaps also beta blockers (another increasingly standard practice in treating heart disease) to those patients for whom there are no counter indications for taking them.

Along with this you would strongly encourage all participants who are not already doing so to adopt a diet that is low in saturated fat. Such encouragement would include referral to a dietitian as you, and some of the patients, are aware that doctors receive very little training in nutrition. The diet would continue to be strongly encouraged throughout the study. Following this, assignment of participants would be randomly made to the control and experimental groups (i.e., placebo and new drug, respectively).

If, however, your primary interest is to "prove" the value of the new drug, then you will not tell any of your subjects to take aspirin or a beta blocker, or strongly encourage them to follow a strict, heart-healthy diet. Rather, you will compare the group taking the drug to a group which takes a placebo, and you would merely advise, not strongly encourage, a diet of 30 percent or less total fat. This way you will maximize the chances that the drug will be found to have positive effects, even though it adds nothing, or may even add a negative element, to what already exists in recommended interventions. It should come to no surprise to readers that it is this design that has become standard in such studies, as we shall see in chapter seven.

Quality versus Quantity of Life

In determining the value of a medical intervention two questions should be asked: "Does it improve the quality of the person's life?" and "Does it extend the person's life?" If it does both, so much the better, if neither, then it should not be invoked. If it does one, but at the expense of the other, then it depends, or should depend on what the person considers of most value. Some believe quality of life is the more important: that a short, sweet life is preferable to one involving more suffering than joy or more confusion than comprehension. Others believe that quantity of life is the only important thing: that life itself, even if in a perpetual coma, is a God-given gift that should not be shortened. We will take the middle course and say that both quantity and quality of life are important and should be measured to determine the value of most, if not all, medical interventions.

Using "end points" to measure quantity of extended life

An "end point" is an outcome that serves to determine the effectiveness of an intervention. Another expression for it is "outcome criterion." However, being that many of the studies in the professional literature use the words "end point" to represent outcome criterion, we may as well get used to it here. The outcomes judged most important to measure are delegated as "main end points." There are usually no more than one or two, one reason being that they are often not independent of each other and statistical analyses lose their power to discern reliable results with each subsequent analysis. Investigators can avoid drawing attention to weaknesses of the experimental intervention by carefully selecting end points.

Surrogate end points are results that are easily obtained and give precise measurements, but which are only indicative, and not definitive of effectiveness. For example, blood cholesterol levels, such as total cholesterol, HDL, and LDL, are all surrogate end points. They are often used in preliminary investigations due to their ease of determination, thus allowing experiments to be done rather quickly on small numbers of subjects. They substitute for waiting long enough to find out if the intervention actually affects the rate of death. The hazard exists that too much faith will be put in the strength of their relationship to actual mortality.

William Silverman[18] provides a graphic example of this hazard in his book, "Where's the Evidence?" An antiarrhythmic drug, flecainide, was found to be very effective in suppressing certain cardiac contractions. On the basis of a presumed connection between these premature cardiac contractions and sudden cardiac death, the FDA adopted the suppression of these premature cardiac contractions as a surrogate end point and permitted the marketing of procaine, and later, a similar drug, encainide. It took eight years of reports of excessive deaths involving the use of these drugs before a properly conducted, multiyear trial found that twice as many patients receiving flecainide or encainide died than did those who received no such drugs. By that time approximately 200,000 patients were taking these drugs, at a conservative estimate of 5,000 deaths per year.

Combined end points, single-cause mortality, and all-cause mortality

For any intervention that is intended to extend life the primary questions are lives truly extended, and, if so, for how long. Any event short of death, no matter how important in itself in other ways, is a surrogate criterion. Thus, just because you have a heart attack does not mean that you are going to die soon, or even sooner than others of your age and sex. In fact, it may serve as a "wake-up call" and get you to change your lifestyle in such a way and to such a degree that you actually live longer than normal. However, death can take a long time to arrive for most of the people in any given study. This makes it difficult to detect any definite difference in the rates of death between two groups of people, even if it exists, until many years have passed. And the longer a study lasts the more expensive it is. Hence, "combined end points" have been invented, combinations of actual deaths and of short-of-death events due to the disease or condition being studied. For example, in one study of a drug for heart disease, fatal and nonfatal myocardial infarctions were combined with unstable angina or sudden cardiac death to make one end point – the primary one.[19] This allows statistically significant differences between the two groups to be found that would otherwise not show up as soon or would not show up at all. However, the most that can be proven then is not really that the intervention is life prolonging, but rather that it reduces certain kinds of heart disease events.

Hence, studies which evaluate the effects of interventions that are intended to be life extending should use **single-cause mortality**, in this case death from coronary disease, as a primary end point. Otherwise, we cannot be sure that the intervention truly is effective in preventing death from the particular disease or condition for which it has been designed. No surrogate end point can substitute for death.

Single-cause mortality pales in significance compared to another end point – **all-cause mortality**. Most of us are more concerned with <u>when</u> we die rather than <u>what</u> we die of. Thus, a treatment that keeps people from dying from heart disease but somehow causes, or does not stop them, from dying of something else a few months later is not of much value. <u>Accordingly, death from any and all causes, often referred to as "all-cause</u>

mortality," should be the other primary end point for any intervention that is to be assessed for its life-extending value. An important advantage of using this as a primary end point is that death itself is easy to determine, whereas death from any particular cause is a matter of diagnostic complexity. We can be sure that someone died but uncertain of what she or he died of, especially if the person suffered from several diseases and perhaps was also suffering from a fall or other trauma.

Using all-cause mortality eliminates a subtle bias factor. If those who do the diagnoses for some reason would prefer that a particular cause of death, say coronary heart disease, be lower in one group, say the experimental drug group, and higher in another group, say the nondrug taking group, then they may consciously or unconsciously lean in the direction that they favor when making the diagnoses. Competent planners of clinical trials try to rule out this type of bias by "blinding" the diagnosticians to which group the subjects are in, but this is not always completely possible. Worse yet, many accepted treatments were never subject to carefully done clinical trials and thus the diagnosed cause of death was definitely susceptible to investigator bias.

Many studies choose single-cause mortality or a combined end point as their sole primary end point. Thus, studies on treatments for heart disease will count only deaths diagnosed as being caused by heart disease, and studies on treatments for breast cancer will measure only the number of deaths diagnosed as caused by breast cancer, etc. This makes it much easier and much less expensive to show positive results from the treatment than when one measures all-cause mortality.

There are several reasons why it is difficult to demonstrate differences in the rate of all-cause mortality. One is that the longer one lives, the more deteriorated all organs of the body become and thus the more prone we are to fall sick of one of many, many different diseases or traumas, all of which "compete" to bring about death. So if one cause is postponed or eliminated, it is likely other things will come to the fore and cause death within a relatively short period of time. Resultantly, it is difficult to change the all-cause death rate and extend life very much unless the intervention prevents death at a relatively early age.[20]

Another factor is that subtle side effects of the intervention may not be noticed during the study or only show up after the study is over - effects which lead to death at a later point. So if you, as an investigator, are interested in showing that an intervention (a drug, surgery, or what have you) extends life without any serious side effects, then you stay away from determining all-cause mortality and all-reported treatment (discussed below). Contrariwise, if you are a recipient of the intervention, you will be much more interested in knowing whether, in fact, your life is likely to be significantly lengthened as a result of the intervention and what quality of life any extension will provide.

A third reason commercial interests would want to avoid using all-cause mortality as a main end point is due to what is called increase in random variation. The difference in deaths between the group treated with the experimental intervention and the control group may be due to many causes, unrelated to the experiment, which accidentally lead to one group suffering more deaths than the other within any given time period. For example, it may just be, simply by luck of the draw that more people died in vehicular accidents in one group than in the other. The only way to rule this out as being due to the experimental intervention is to increase the number of subjects or to lengthen the period of observation. This increases the cost of the experiment. However, it also increases the reliability of the results in terms of whether or not the experimental intervention truly is beneficial.

Quality of life and how it is measured: Quality-Adjusted Life Years (QALYs)

The quality of the life that is extended is the other major concern in any life-extending treatment. Some individuals would consider that the primary concern. They would be more concerned with dying from a disease associated with drawn-out disability and suffering, than dying sooner from heart disease or other cause not typically associated with such consequences.

Yet, among the missing components in almost all follow-ups is systematic measurement of quality of life. **Fortunately, a measure has been developed that takes into account both the length of the extension of life and the quality of the remaining years. It is referred to as the Quality-Adjusted Life Year or "QALY."** There are many formulas for this measure, and other names, and a lot of discussion as to which components should be in it and how they should be measured, but the concept itself is generally accepted.[21,22] The measure can be used in determining the relative costs of competing interventions, and, in fact, was devised for this purpose.[23,24]

Doing a good job of gathering data for this sort of instrument requires recording two aspects of postintervention quality of life. One is how people feel about the quality of their life. The other aspect is determination of the symptoms they have experienced, especially those for which they required treatment. For studies in which the intervention is a continuing one, such as a drug one takes indefinitely, the study should last for a long time. If the intervention is "acute," such as one-time surgery, the length of the study could be shorter. The assessment of both quality of life and of symptoms requiring treatment should be done regularly throughout the length of the study, being careful not to favor sampling of times when the patients are apt to feel at their "best."

Single-cause, all-cause, and all-reported treatments

Single-cause treatment refers to treatment that was given as a result of a single cause, whether it be a disease or a trauma. Coronary bypass surgery, for example, would be a treatment "caused by" coronary disease (actually this surgery is an optional treatment, but so are most treatments). It is important to determine if, and by how much, an intervention - a drug, for example - intended to reduce the effects of coronary disease reduced the treatments and costs due to such disease. If it didn't reduce such treatment or only reduced it an insignificant amount, then the intervention would not be of any value, unless it somehow managed to extend life anyway.

All-cause treatment refers to treatments of illness or disability of any kind. One does not have to know what, exactly, is causing the problem to know that there is a problem which resulted in treatment -- be it for headache, dizziness, nausea, movement pain of some kind, or what have you. Thus, like all-cause mortality, it is independent of diagnostic accuracy. As such, it should be a main criteria for measuring the effectiveness of an intervention, especially one that is intended as an ameliorative treatment rather than as a life-extender. It, like all-cause mortality, will accurately express the fact that not suffering from one disease does not exclude you from suffering from others. It will also express the side effects of any treatment.

There is a practical problem, however, in attempting to measure all-cause treatment: it is hard, if not impossible, to obtain all the data. For one thing, people often go to several different practitioners and purchase a host of different remedies for their various ailments, and it may be difficult for them to keep track of all their sufferings and the treatments for them. For another, they may not want to divulge some of the ailments which they developed, such as sexual problems.

However, this does not rule out asking subjects what other medical problems and treatments they remember having and recording them, and then add this to what can be found out from other sources. This would more thoroughly detect any side effects of the experimental treatment, especially subtle ones. **One could call this "all-reported treatment."** Anything that appears to be significant should be revealed in publicized reports so it can be followed up in other studies and alert clinicians to looking for such problems in the patients who have received the prescribed intervention.

Early cessation of the study

Another practice that can bias the findings is to stop the experiment at the point if and when the results become statistically significant rather than at the planned final date. This practice allows studies to be terminated early when the experimental treatment is found to be clearly causing more harm than good. It is also used when it definitely is more beneficial than the control treatment, normally the usual treatment for the malady in question. The problem is how to determine when something is "clearly" causing more harm or more good. A certain level of statistical significance often becomes the criterion. The results are calculated at various intervals and at any point that this level is reached between the groups, a decision can be made to terminate the study. This practice has the side effect of lowering the expense of the study. However, statistical significance is not equivalent to real, practical significance. It can be reached simply by having large numbers of subjects, even though the actual difference may be small and of little clinical significance. Stopping a study early because of clinically small, but statistically significant findings that support the experimental intervention, precludes the discovery of unanticipated serious side effects that take additional time to manifest themselves. If the study were continued, the results might actually reverse themselves.

If there is a prejudgment-bias to find the experimental intervention superior to that of the comparison treatment, this can show up in decisions to stop the trial early. Silverman[18] provides an example of this: a clinical trial found the death rate for hospital-treated patients suffering from heart disease to be slightly higher than those who were treated at home. Someone reversed the figures and showed them to a proponent of hospital treatment, who then immediately demanded that the trial be terminated, finding it unethical to continue to treat patients at home. However, when the correct results were then shown to him, the physician did not find it unethical to continue the study.

Missing long-term effects

In dealing with humans whose average life span averages from around 70 to 80 years in First World countries, it is important to measure the effects of long-term treatments. Surgical interventions, for example, may weaken organs or other parts of the body in ways which are not noticed until years later when the person is weakened by illness or age. Drugs which are to be taken indefinitely may slowly induce changes which can lead to cancer or other maladies, or they may have subtle psychological effects which are prone to be attributed to situational factors, other illnesses, or to chronic stress. Only truly long-term, comprehensive observation can pick up such effects.

For example, halcyon was used for years as a sleep-aiding drug before it was found that it caused amnesia and other side effects. The fact that this was discovered at all is somewhat of a wonder given the effectiveness of the voluntary reporting system that is in place. It has been estimated that only about 10 percent of adverse reactions get reported after drugs have been released for marketing.[25]

From our review of hundreds of studies, the effects of many medical interventions are often not measured past the point of leaving the hospital or for a few months to a couple of years. Five-year follow-ups of any kind are rare. In fact, they have become identified as being long-term. Truly long-term follow-ups which can pick up on subtle side effects are virtually nonexistent. Requiring the determination of all-cause mortality as a main end point for supposed life-extending interventions would promote longer-term follow-ups.

We shall return to these topics in later chapters when we apply the Proposed Standards to specific procedures. The next chapter concerns the next stage in research, the presentation and publication of the results.

PROPOSED STANDARDS FOR RESEARCH DESIGN

III **No "straw men" comparisons.** **Trial studies should be designed in such a way as to compare the experimental procedures and products to one or more robust alternative treatments, if such exist, and not to weak versions of them. When the alternative treatment is "standard medical practice," it should not be some weak version of it, but rather one which the physicians and other personnel are carefully instructed in what is recommended practice.**

If this standard is not observed, it is impossible to determine how much, if any, the intervention adds to what can already be accomplished by following recommended practice.

IV   In any nonpreliminary study, use both single-cause and all-cause
     mortality as main end points in any intervention that purports to
     be life extending. Do not settle for surrogate end points, even if
     combined with a mortality end point, since this negates the value
     of the end point.

        Surrogate end points have been found to be inadequate and to
     lead to adoption of intervention with unknown, even deadly
     effects. Hence they are to be avoided as main end points in any
     final assessments of life-extending interventions. Combining
     them with mortality in a main end point only obscures the
     results as to actual effects on mortality and lends itself to abuse
     by those who wish to promote a particular intervention when the
     surrogate end point(s) are more promising than the mortality
     end points.

V   Use all-reported treatment in determining any change in quality
     of life due to interventions that are intended to be primarily
     ameliorative in nature.

        To truly determine the degree, extent, and nature of side
     effects of any intervention, it is insufficient to merely look at the
     effects that are obviously connected to it, such as the effects on
     the morbidity of that particular disease, since other disease
     processes may be triggered by the intervention. Also, trauma
     could result, such as a fall or an automobile accident caused by
     dizziness which is a side effect of the drug. Hence, it is necessary
     to determine, as much as possible, all the postintervention
     treatments that patients report or their records reveal, i.e., all-
     reported treatment.

VI   Use all-cause mortality and all-reported treatment in the
     calculation of Quality-Adjusted Life Years gained.

        Only a full accounting of all intervention effects can result in
     an accurate measuring of QALYs.

> **VII** **No early termination of studies for less than truly good reasons.** Ongoing studies should not be cut short before the full term solely for the reason that a statistically significant result has been reached for a main end point. They should be stopped only if the proportional difference is obviously of clinical significance (for example, the incidence of permanent disability or the number of deaths are clearly higher in one group and there seems to be no other plausible explanation for that).
>
> Stopping a trial early is a judgment call that lends itself to bias in favor of what the investigators had hoped to prove was true. It stops short any correction to the results that would occur if there were a reversal of the findings in the later stage of the study.

References

[1] Waughman PG, Porter R J (1992). Mechanisms of interaction between industry and the academic medical center. In: Porter RJ, Malone TE, eds. *Biomedical research: collaboration and conflict of interest*. Baltimore: The Johns Hopkins University Press: 93-118.

[2] Garrow J (1994). Sometimes consultancies cannot be disclosed. *BMJ* 308: 471.

[3] Campbell EG, Lewis KS, Blumenthal D (1998). Looking a gift horse in the mouth. *JAMA* 279: 995-99.

[4] Rifkin J (1998). *The biotech century*. New York: Jeremy P Tarcher / Putman: 56.

[5] Cooper T, Novitch M (1992). The research needs of industry: working together with academia and with the federal government. In: Porter RJ, Malone TE, eds. *Biomedical research: collaboration and conflict of interest*. Baltimore: The Johns Hopkins University Press: 187-98.

[6] Witt MD, Goslin LO (1994). Conflict of interest dilemmas in biomedical research. *JAMA* 271: 547-51.

[7] Nightingale St L (1998). From the Food and Drug Administration. *JAMA* 279: 984.

[8] Josefson D (1998). FDA rules that researchers will have to disclose financial interest. *BMJ* 316: 493.

[9] Porter RJ (1992). Conflicts of interest in research: the fundamentals. In: Porter and Malone (pp. 121-34). See note one.

[10] Davidson RA (1986). Source of funding and outcome of clinical trials. *J Gen Intern Med* 3:155-58.

[11] Friedberg M, Saffran B, et al. (1999). Evaluation of conflict of interest in economical analyses of new drugs used in oncology. *JAMA* 282: 1453-57.

[12] Stelfox H T, Grace C, et al. (1998). Conflict of interest in the debate over calcium-channel antagonists. *N Engl J Med* 338: 101-06.

[13] Angell M (2000). Is academic medicine for sale? *N Engl J Med* 342: 1516-18.

[14] Bodenheimer T (2000). Uneasy alliance: clinical investigators and the pharmaceutical industry. *N Engl J Med* 342: 1539-44.

[15] Chen PS Jr (1992). The National Institutes of Health and Its Interactions with Industry. In: Porter and Malone (pp. 199-221). See note one above.

[16] Vaughan CC, Smith BLR, Porter RJ (1992). The contribution of biomedical science and technology to U.S. economic competitiveness. In: Porter RJ, Malone TE, eds. *Biomedical research: collaboration and conflict of interest.* Baltimore: The Johns Hopkins University Press: 57-76.

[17] Council on Scientific Affairs and Council on Ethical and Judicial Affairs (1990). *JAMA* 263: 2790-93.

[18] Silverman W (1999). *Where's the evidence?* New York: Oxford University Press.

[19] Downs JR, Clearfield M, et al. (1998). Primary prevention of acute coronary events with Lovastatin in men and women with average cholesterol levels. *JAMA* 279: 1615-22.

[20] The limits of life (January-February, 1991). *Hastings Center Report*: 48.

[21] Canadian Coordinating Office for Health Technology Assessment (November, 1997). *Guidelines for economic evaluation of pharmaceuticals*: Ottawa, Ontario K2C 3V4, Canada. www.ccohta.ca

[22] Briggs A, Gray A (1999). Handling uncertainty in economic evaluations of healthcare interventions. *BMJ* 319: 635-38.

[23] Drummond MF, Richardson WF, et al. (1997). Users' guide to the medical literature: How to use an article on economic analysis of clinical practice. *JAMA* 277: 1552-57.

[24] Greenhalgh T (1997). Papers that tell you what things cost (economic analyses). *BMJ* 315: 596-99.

[25] Pirmohamed M, Breckenbridge AM, et al. (1998). Adverse drug reactions. *BMJ* 316: 1295-98.

Chapter Four

Disseminating the Results

Andrew Thompson, Matthias Egger

The role of the public and professional media in medicine cannot be underestimated. What is said, seen, or heard on a mass basis has tremendous impact on what treatments are demanded and prescribed. It also has substantial impact on the stock prices of companies who offer the product or an essential portion of the procedure involved, such as the diagnostic testing kit or the medical apparatus.[1] Release of promising results of incomplete or preliminary studies via statements made in conferences attended by reporters, by official press releases, and by publication in professional journals can persuade politicians, funding services, practitioners, and the general public to demand that the treatment be offered immediately to all who might benefit from it.

Such publicity can be so powerful in its effect that planned research to determine the value of the experimental treatment in a more complete, thorough, and reliable manner, cannot be done. This may be because either the physicians refuse to administer the "old," supposedly inferior treatment or potential participants refuse to risk being assigned to it rather than to the new "wonder" treatment.

HOW CLINICAL RESEARCH IS CONDUCTED

The "Phase Process" for the evaluation of new treatments (see Table 1) is designed to optimize the chances that any positive results of the experimental intervention will be spotted. It also enhances the probability that "false positives" will emerge, results that look promising but are later found not to be so after more thorough studies are conducted.

A. Thompson and N.J. Temple (eds.), Ethics, Medical Research, and Medicine, 41–58.

Table 1. **The Phase Process of testing new drugs in human beings**

Phase I trial	A trial involving the first application of a new treatment to humans and conducted to provide information on metabolism, pharmacological action, and safety of a drug. Phase I trials are usually uncontrolled trials, without a concurrently enrolled comparison group. They assess surrogate end points.
Phase II trials	The main purpose of phase II trials is to provide preliminary information on the efficacy of the drug and added information on safety. The study design may include a control treatment and random assignment to the treatment groups. The study assesses surrogate end points or clinical events.
Phase III trials	Usually the final stage in relation to a new drug application, phase III trials are concerned with assessment of dosage effects, efficacy, and safety and aimed at providing information for labeling in relation to use in the clinical setting. Usually designed to include a control treatment and random assignment to treatment. May assess surrogate endpoints or clinical events.
Phase IV trials	Trials performed after approval of the drug by licensing bodies, typically performed under circumstances approximating real-world conditions and usually with a clinical event as the primary outcome and long-term follow-up. The effectiveness and safety of a given drug is compared with a control treatment, usually in a randomized trial.
Postmarketing surveillance	Any system implemented after approval of a drug or device to provide ongoing information on the use of the drug in relation to approved indications and on uncommon clinical adverse effects. The surveillance usually involves surveys and observational study designs.

Adapted from Meinert[2]

The last and most important stages, large randomized phase III/IV trials, may never be completed if the results of smaller studies are publicized. If these results are described as showing clear superiority of the new treatment, recruitment of new subjects for large phase III/IV trials may become problematic since potential subjects will refuse to take the risk that they might be randomly assigned to the "inferior" treatment. Physicians may also refuse to give patients what they now think is likely to be the less effective conventional treatment. Instead, they will recommend the new, unproven, and probably more expensive treatment.

For phase III trials, the primary end point should ideally be a clinical event that is relevant to the patient and not a laboratory measurement or clinical sign. For example, it is insufficient to show that a drug lowers serum cholesterol levels or reduces blood pressure. The demonstration that it prevents heart attacks and reduces mortality from cardiovascular disease is what counts. In practice, laboratory measurements or physical signs are, however, often used as a substitute ('surrogate end point') for a clinically meaningful end point to reduce costs and shorten the duration of phase III trials.[3]

We shall go into this in more detail in our discussion of breast and prostate cancer but shall touch upon examples now which illustrate that the results from the initial phases of the evaluation of new treatments are prone to being distorted and misinterpreted.

AUTOLOGOUS BONE MARROW TRANSPLANTATION FOR BREAST CANCER

Autologous Bone Marrow Transplantation (ABMT) is a method whereby transplantation of a patient's own bone marrow is used to protect her from the otherwise lethal doses of chemotherapy designed to combat breast cancer. Phase I studies indicated that generally unhealthy patients and those who responded poorly to initial chemotherapy did very poorly with ABMT. Thus in phase II studies, ABMT was performed primarily on women who responded well to initial chemotherapy and were healthier than others who had similar states of advanced cancer. The average length of survival of this select group of relatively healthy ABMT recipients was then compared to the average length of survival of all women with similar stages of advanced cancer, including the relatively unhealthy ones. As would be expected, the initially healthier-than-average ABMT group survived somewhat longer.[4]

These distorted results were released and the media picked up on it, describing ABMT as "a magic bullet."[5] As a result, breast cancer became the most common disease for which transplant therapy was given in the 1990s.[6] The public, including physicians, were persuaded that a new, effective treatment had been found for breast cancer. Thousands of women worldwide underwent transplant therapy, often as part of routine medical care. Patients have sued insurers who have refused to pay for this expensive treatment, and courts have awarded damages to some of the plaintiffs, and forced some U.S. states to require insurers to provide such coverage.[7-8] Furthermore, a treatment supposed to be reserved for women in the last stages of breast cancer has been demanded by and administered to those with less advanced stages of the disease.[9]

As a result it has become difficult to find sufficient physicians and patients to participate in the trials with clinical end points which require random assignment of eligible patients to ABMT or to conventional treatment.[4] Physicians and patients believe in ABMT and refuse to participate in any study in which some patients would "risk" being assigned to conventional chemotherapy. A number of trials have nevertheless been set up and the preliminary results from four trials indicate that high dose chemotherapy followed by ABMT does not significantly improve survival.[10] These studies will continue for another two to four years. A fifth trial, from South Africa, did find a reduced mortality after five years of follow-up[11]; however, an on-site review of the study found inconsistencies between the patient records and the data presented at international meetings and Werner Bezwoda, the primary investigator, recently admitted to scientific misconduct.[6] Given the lack of persuasive data demonstrating superior effectiveness of this very toxic therapy, the American Society of Clinical Oncology now recommends that high dose chemotherapy followed by ABMT for breast cancer should only be performed in the context of a high quality clinical trial.[12]

SUPPRESSION OF IRREGULAR HEARTBEAT AFTER MYOCARDIAL INFARCTION AND THE HAZARD OF SETTLING FOR A SURROGATE END POINT

Irregular heartbeat due to ventricular arrhythmia is a well-known risk factor in patients with heart disease. The risk of death, in particular sudden death, is substantially increased in heart patients with ventricular arrhythmia.[13] Three new drugs (flecainide, encainide, and moricizine) that were found to effectively suppress irregular heartbeats were licensed by the Food and Drug Administration (FDA) for use in patients with severe, life-threatening, or **severely** symptomatic arrhythmias. Once a drug is approved for one indication, doctors have much latitude in prescribing it for other uses. And, indeed, this is what happened with these drugs. Thousands of patients with heart disease and **asymptomatic** arrhythmias eventually took these drugs over extended periods of time to prevent sudden death despite the fact no trials had been done in this group and the drugs were not approved for this indication.[14] The Cardiac Arrhythmia Suppression Trial

(CAST) was finally set up to examine whether the three drugs would reduce mortality in patients with asymptomatic ventricular arrhythmia who had had a heart attack. The results were startling: the flecainide and encainide arms had to be stopped because mortality was almost three times higher with these drugs than with placebo.[14] The final results of the CAST trials showed that mortality was also increased with moricizine.[15]

This is a classic example demonstrating the unreliability of surrogate end points, but many other examples exist.[16] It also shows that drug companies do not have to subject their products to large clinical trials and wait for approval for other applications once a drug has been approved for one application. In this situation, the media often become a powerful ally of the pharmaceutical industry by enthusiastically and uncritically reporting on the apparent benefits in unapproved applications, thereby raising demand and sales.[17]

Knowing the credulity and susceptibility of patients and physicians to announcements of newfound "miracle treatments," it is irresponsible for those who have access to such preliminary results to release them to representatives of the mass media where news of killer bacteria and miraculous therapies compete with murders, ecological catastrophes, and the life events of the glitterati.[18]

WHAT GETS INTO PRINT? THE ROLE OF SCIENTIFIC JOURNALS

Bad news is not popular: discrediting or ignoring the messenger rather than accepting the message is as frequent in the field of medical research as in other spheres of human endeavor. Scientific articles that indicate that experimental drugs don't work, that surgery creates more problems than it cures, or that diagnostic technology leads to more false diagnoses than correct are less likely to be get published than studies reporting 'positive' results. Hypothetically, with a putative therapy that has no actual effect on a disease, it is possible that studies which suggest a beneficial treatment effect will be published, while an equal mass of data pointing the other way will remain unpublished. In the field of cancer chemotherapy such **publication bias** has indeed been demonstrated by comparing the results from studies identified in a literature search with those contained in an international trials registry.[19] Registration generally takes place before completion of the study and the criteria that qualify for registration are exclusively based on design features. The studies enlisted in a register are therefore likely to constitute a more representative sample of all the studies that have been performed in a given area than a sample of published studies. This has been shown with advanced ovarian cancer where the analysis of published randomized clinical trials indicated considerably better survival with combination chemotherapy as compared to alkylating agent monotherapy. However, an analysis of the registered trials failed to confirm this.[19]

THE IMPACT OF STATISTICAL SIGNIFICANCE

Several studies have investigated the importance of publication bias in the medical literature by following up research proposals approved by ethics committees or institutional review boards.[20] The factors associated with publication or nonpublication of results could thus be examined. For example, of 285 studies approved by the Central Oxford Research Ethics Committee between 1984 and 1987, which had been completed and analyzed, only 138 (48 percent) had been published by 1990.[21] Studies with statistically significant results were more likely to have been published than those with nonsignificant results, regardless of the quality of the research. A review of five such studies showed that this is a consistent finding: the odds of publication were three times greater if the results were statistically significant.[20] Studies with statistically significant results are also published more rapidly whereas 'negative' studies, if published at all, are published with considerable delay. Among proposals submitted to the Royal Prince Alfred Hospital Ethics Committee in Sydney, around 85 percent of studies with significant results had been published after 10 years but only 65 percent of studies with null results.[22] The median time to publication was 4.8 years for studies with significant results and 8.0 years for studies with null results. By that time the latter studies had probably lost most, if not all, of whatever corrective influence they might have had. Such *time lag bias* was also shown for AIDS trials.[23]

The number of times a published study is cited in subsequent publications is an indication of its impact. Studies with negative results have been shown to have less impact than studies reporting statistically significant results (*citation bias*). For example, in the field of cholesterol lowering, trials which are supportive of a beneficial effect were cited more frequently than unsupportive trials (the mean annual number of citations was 40 versus 7), regardless of the size and quality of the studies involved.[24] Finally, studies with significant results are more likely to lead to multiple publications and presentations.[21] The production of duplicate publications from single studies can lead to bias in a number of ways (*multiple publication bias*).[25] The inclusion of duplicated data in reviews may lead to overestimation of treatment effects, as recently demonstrated for trials of ondansetron for prevention of postoperative nausea and vomiting.[26] It is not always obvious that multiple publications come from a single study, since examples exist where two articles reporting the same trial do not even share a single common author.[25,26]

A PARTIAL REMEDY: REGISTRATION OF CLINICAL TRIALS

A partial remedy for this situation has been proposed. It is to require that all planned clinical trials be entered on a common, publicly accessible, international registry -- whether or not they get published.[27,28,29] This way members of evidence-based medicine, meta-analysts and other reviewers of studies, and anyone else with an interest or a concern could access the true range of information in a given area. The Cochrane Collaboration, an international, nonprofit organization, offers such a registry. In response to requests by this organization, one company, Glaxo Wellcome, has agreed to register its clinical trials worldwide, and another, Schering Health Care, will put information on its ongoing controlled trials in the Cochrane Controlled Trials Register.[28,30] It is to be hoped that the other pharmaceutical firms will follow suit.

THE ROLE OF EDITORS AND REVIEWERS AND FINANCIAL CONFLICTS OF INTEREST

Editors serve as the primary gatekeepers in the process of deciding if an article should be published at all, or only with alterations, or rejected outright. In a peer review journal they will turn to experts in the field which the article covers to aid in this decision. If either these reviewers or the editors can expect to benefit or lose financially, depending on whether the article is published or published in an altered form, then they may favor some articles and not others. Recognition of these facts has led recently to some journals adopting financial disclosure requirements from not only the paper's authors, but also of prospective reviewers, and in some cases also of the journal's editors. The International Committee of Medical Journal Editors "has identified financial relations with industry (for example, employment, consultancies, stock ownership, honoraria, expert testimony), either directly or through immediate family, as the most important conflicts of interest." It furthermore "considers that the manner in which authors, reviewers, and editors deal with such conflicts can affect in part the credibility of published articles in scientific journals."[31]

However, this is a disputed point, and some argue that there are other factors that are more important potential conflicts, such as intellectual persuasion, academic competition, and personal relationships. Also, that it is sometimes impossible to find a competent reviewer, or author, or editor, who does not have a financial conflict of interest.

We decided to sample the water in this area and sent out a brief questionnaire to the editors of eleven prominent medical journals. Four were British and seven were American journals; some were general medical journals, while others specialized in internal medicine, cancer, or cardiology. We asked about their policies for their editorial staff. Nine of the eleven responded, some after a reminder letter. Only three required disclosure of possible conflicts of interest. Only one required divestment of any financial conflict, although two said they would, in some cases, if known. Only two automatically precluded editors from the decision making process who had a conflict, but two others said they would in some cases. What is perhaps most interesting is that two said they were developing a formal policy to cover these issues.

The *New England Journal of Medicine* (*NEJM*) is the most stringent in this matter. Its ten-year old policy requires full disclosure from all editors and divestment of any financial conflicts of interest. It has also attempted to get full disclosure from its authors and peer reviewers, with mixed success. After the *Los Angeles Times* published two articles revealing that *NEJM* authors of reviews "had financial links to drug companies that sold products they were writing about" the *NEJM* did its own review and found 19 rule-breaking articles and blamed the mistakes on a loophole in their policy. The authors were not directly reimbursed or supported by the drug companies, but the institutions they worked for were. This loophole is to be closed.[32]

THE ROLE OF INDUSTRY-SPONSORED STUDIES

Studies have indicated that the source of funding is associated with publication or nonpublication, independent of study results. Studies sponsored by the pharmaceutical industry were less likely to be published than those supported by the government or by voluntary organizations. Investigators assert that data management by these companies is a reason for nonpublication.[33,21] This is in agreement with a review of publications of clinical trials. This separated them into those that were sponsored by the pharmaceutical industry and those supported by other means.[34] The results of 89 percent of published trials supported by industry favored the new therapy, as compared to 61 percent of the other trials. Similar results have been reported from an overview of trials of nonsteroidal anti-inflammatory drugs.[35] The implication is that the pharmaceutical industry has blocked the publication of negative studies which it has funded.

Another source of bias in the publishing of the results of trials is that drug companies sometimes offer investigators the assistance of professional ghost writers.[36] It seems unlikely that such assistance would be impartial.

HOW THE RESULTS ARE PRESENTED

In this world no one has enough time to read everything one "should" read, much less read it from start to finish, and even more rarely to make a thorough analysis of the methodology and data analysis in order to draw independent conclusions from the basic data. We have become an audience of "skimmers," with the result that many read only the abstract of most scientific articles and possibly the concluding remarks, or perhaps only the title and first few lines. If any of these parts are misrepresentative of the article as a whole, we walk away with a false impression of its contents. Thus, for authors to deliberately or carelessly misrepresent the contents in their abstracts, conclusions, titles, or introductory lines is inappropriate. It is also inadequate to deliberately or carelessly make it difficult to comprehend and challenge the conclusions of the article by omitting selected data or explanations as to how it was arrived at, or, in general, to write in such a murky fashion that it is difficult to impossible for even dedicated and expert readers to figure out exactly what was done. Although initiatives such as the Consolidated Standards of Reporting Clinical Trials (CONSORT)[37] should improve this situation, the reporting and conduct of clinical trials is grossly inadequate at present.[38]

Results in the abstract and in the article itself are usually presented in terms of statistics. We all know that "statistics can lie" - that is, they can be accurate in themselves yet lead to false conclusions. Researchers and other members of the medical industry are among those who commonly use statistics in this manner. The most common way in which this is done is to use "relative difference" rather than "absolute difference" as a means of reporting the results of an experimental treatment.

For example, the West of Scotland Coronary Prevention Study (WOSCOPS) of pravastatin, a cholesterol lowering drug, in men with hypercholesterolemia but no history of heart disease reported a relative reduction in the mortality from coronary heart disease of 30 percent and a reduction in total mortality of 22 percent over five years.[39] Surveys among patients[40], general practitioners[41,42], and doctors in teaching hospitals[43] have all shown that people are more likely to believe an intervention is desirable when effectiveness data is presented as a relative risk reduction rather than when data from the same studies is presented in absolute terms. This is hardly surprising: in WOSCOPS coronary mortality was reduced from 1.7 percent to 1.2 percent and total mortality from 4.1 percent to 3.2 percent.[44] A headline reading "0.5 percent advantage for new drug for preventing death from coronary heart disease" is not likely to be selected by the editor. What is more directly relevant to us is that if the drug's effectiveness were to be described in this way, patients may very well forego taking the drug, especially if they would have to take it lifelong and it may have quite unpleasant or even dangerous side effects. In the case of WOSCOPS it can be calculated that 200 men with no prior heart disease will have to swallow 358,000 tablets over five years to save one of them from dying from coronary heart disease.[44]

A reverse phenomenon occurs when it comes to describing the adverse side effects of an intervention. American physicians use the Physicians Desk Reference (PDR) to find out about adverse effects. The PDR descriptions are written by the drug companies that market the drugs. Whereas pharmaceutical company brochures describe positive treatment effects in relative statistics, the adverse effects in the PDR are in terms of absolute risk reductions. As a result physicians are likely to use the relative risk provided them in reporting the potentially positive aspects of a proposed treatment and absolute risk in describing the potentially negative results. For example, "Less than five percent suffer an adverse side effect from this drug treatment, but it offers a 50 percent chance of improvement over no treatment." Such a statement could actually mean that there is a greater chance of an adverse side effect than of a benefit!

For those who are determined to promote a particular intervention, there are many other ways to make the intervention appear in a favorable light. For example, most studies allow for a variety of statistical methods for analyzing the results. Authors can choose the combination that best presents the actual results or one, perhaps less justifiable on mathematical grounds, that provides what the authors want the study to show. Choosing the latter, of course, is unethical.[45] An increasingly popular method for statistically combining studies, meta-analysis, provides summary results in a given area. However, there is considerable danger that meta-analyses of studies of doubtful quality, of heterogeneous studies or studies affected by publication bias will produce spurious results.[46,20] In other words, "junk in, junk out." Sometimes just leaving out or including one large study or one study with "extreme" results, can make a significant difference. With enough chutzpah a creative writer can pretty much "prove" anything.

HOW DARE YOU? HARASSMENT OF INVESTIGATORS WHO PUBLISH INDUSTRY-UNFRIENDLY RESULTS

Hardiness is required by authors and institutions who dare to publish industry-unfriendly results, as illustrated by the following case histories.[47] Researchers at the University of Washington in the USA published several studies that questioned the value of spinal-fusion surgery and wrote guidelines for managing acute back problems that would reduce its use. The federally supported Agency for Health Care Policy and Research funded the studies and the guideline development process, the researchers were thus independent of funding from profit-making sources. The North American Spine Association, which represents the interests of neurosurgeons and other professionals providing spine care responded by successfully lobbying the House of Representatives to withdraw funding from the agency. Strenuous efforts were required in the Senate to partially restore this funding but the authority to develop guidelines was taken away.

In the second case investigators and inquiry boards bore the brunt of the attack. Investigators from a group health cooperative published a study that cast doubt on the value of diagnostic tests for chemical sensitivity, tests that are used to support disability and liability claims. Plaintiffs' attorneys, advocacy organizations for people with chemical sensitivity, and representatives of immunologic-testing laboratories instituted a range of harassing actions. These included "multiple complaints of scientific misconduct to the sponsoring institutions and the federal Office of Research Integrity, requests to the medical disciplinary board of Washington State that investigators' licenses be revoked, and distribution of materials at scientific meetings that accused investigators of fraud and conspiracy."

As a result of these actions the investigators had to undergo separate inquiries by five different institutions. None of these inquiries found a basis for a full-scale investigation but all of them were extended by the "'outsiders' relentless use of procedures designed primarily to deal with internal whistle-blowers and disputes within research groups." Inquiries that normally require resolution within 30 days lasted more than 13 months.

In the third case investigators and their host university presented a study that threatened to undermine the prescription and sale of certain drugs. The study indicated that short-acting calcium-channel blockers which were used to treat patients with hypertension were associated with a 60 percent increase in myocardial infarctions.[48] It was far from a conclusive study but front-page stories tended to treat it as such. The predictable result was that concerned patients and physicians flooded the investigators with calls. One drug manufacturer went much further. Using the Freedom of Information Act, it requested <u>all</u> records relating to the study, including not only all the data and analysis of the study itself but all minutes of meetings and notes of the investigators and all documentation by any oversight committee both inside and outside the university. The company only withdrew its request after several months of negotiation with the university and the investigators. Academic consultants to companies who manufacture calcium-channel blockers publicly questioned the integrity of the investigators. These consultants usually did not identify their industry connection. Nor did a mass mailing to the same effect to physicians indicate that pharmaceutical companies supported its distribution.

The net effect of such actions is to make funding sources, host institutions, and investigators think twice before conducting research that does not have a more than even chance of producing industry-friendly results.

BUYING EDITORIALS

There are still other ethically suspect ways to manipulate public or professional opinion. Suppose that, despite all the commercial firm's efforts to the contrary, some diagnostic procedure or treatment is called into question in the public media. What kind of damage control measure is available to them? Perhaps the best kind, from their point of view, is to have reputable experts, supposedly unbiased in that they have no obvious ties to industry, make public statements defending the practice. But how to recruit such experts?

One way is to write a less than kosher editorial for them and then pay them for editing it and submitting it to a suggested outlet. It is a common practice for a pharmaceutical company to employ a public relations firm, that, in turn, approaches a respected scholar-scientist and asks the expert to submit an editorial to a professional journal, a popular press magazine, or a newspaper about some current issue of concern to the company. A draft of the editorial, composed by a professional writer, is given to the expert to ease the burden of writing and a generous check is also provided.[49]

This practice has become so prevalent that some journals, such as the major British medical journals, *BMJ* and *Lancet*, require those who submit editorial statements to reveal any financial arrangements that might have influenced them and then publish the information with the article. It is to be hoped that all medical journals will adopt this practice. If the experts were ethical, they would refuse such offers, or, providing they substantially agree with the proposed commentary, they might submit it to the media — but only with a statement fully declaring their relationship with the drug company, and they would require that this disclosure be included. That is, they would take the risk that the editorial would not be published, that they would not be paid, and if it were published, its impact would be reduced. They might also lose out on the opportunity for other such lucrative assignments along with the public or professional recognition of their expertise. To be truly ethical, they would not accept any money in the first place but would instead offer to pay the ghost writer and/or the company for their contribution.

One possible reason for the receptivity of the popular media to medical "advances" is that this is perhaps the only arena in which good news predominates -- and this makes it immensely appealing to the public. Much of the rest of the serious news that is reported is of murders, disasters, wars, and political chicanery -- none of which is very cheering. In one way it would be a shame to deprive people of the myth that medicine is continually making dramatic discoveries that are going to give everyone (in the First World) perfect health and a long life. But this myth is destructively demanding of resources needed elsewhere and it is irresponsible for medical researchers or other professionals to deliberately promote it.

Proposed Standards on Publication

VIII	All clinical trials should be registered in an easily accessible, public, international registry. Reviewers and those who wish to conduct meta-analyses or other aggregate analyses on studies need to identify those trials that led to multiple publications. Information about trials that were not published or completed would also provide useful information for other overview purposes.

IX   Disclosure, Both the funding source(s) for any paper and any financial ties to commercial firms of all investigators in any study should be disclosed to potential publishers and, if the paper is published, this information should also be divulged to readers in a prominent place.

Without such information editors and reviewers, and later the intended readers, are not in a position to judge for themselves the likelihood of commercial bias in the design or write-up of the paper. There are many other kinds of biases, such as favoritism of certain academic institutions, theories, and types of research, but this one is more powerful than others due to its pervasiveness in First World societies where most medical research is done.

X   All major players in the publishing process -- reviewers, editors, and any others who have a say in the final judgement in the acceptance of a paper or book for publication should:

A.   Disclose any financial conflict of interest that might affect their judgement on the decision. This would include any occasional or continuing consultancy or other employment, paid presentations, expense covered trips to conferences, and stock holdings of themselves or family members.

B.   In addition, reviewers should be selected who do not have any such conflict of interest.

C.   Editors, being the primary gatekeepers of the publishing world, should divest themselves of conflicting financial interests, and failing that, withdraw from the decision making process on any submitted paper in which they have a financial interest.

XI	In the abstract or any other prominent place where statistical results are reported, the results between the intervention and the nonintervention group(s) should be expressed primarily in absolute terms, not in terms of relative reductions in risks. Alternative absolute risk-derived measures, such as Number Needed to Treat (NNT), would also be appropriate for prominent placement. Relative-risk reduction, while perhaps necessary or useful for statistical manipulations or comparisons, is a misleading statistic for most readers and for the mass media. It provides an exaggerated impression of the efficacy of an intervention.

XII	No industry-affiliated ghost writers. Assistance from ghost writers for research articles, editorials, and commentaries — either in professional journals or intended for the mass media — should be acknowledged and/or otherwise compensated. Offers from commercial interests to supply writing assistance should be rejected.

XIII	Unbiased publication of all worthy studies and commentaries. Medical journals and other professional publications should institute procedures to insure that articles which are promotive of new products or procedures do not receive more favorable treatment, such as better chance of publication or quicker publication, than those that are critical of products or procedures. This would mean, for example, that papers that claim statistically significant results would not be more likely to be published or published any sooner than papers that find that the intervention does not show any statistically significant advantage over the comparison treatment, or lack of treatment. Also, the editors should critically review all articles submitted for publication to insure that the titles, abstracts, presentation of results, and citation of relevant literature do not distort the likely impact of the article in favor of a commercial or institutional interest.

References

[1] Ferguson JR (1997). Biomedical research and insider trading. *N Engl J Med* 337: 631-34.

[2] Meinert CL (1995). *Clinical Trials Dictionary*. Baltimore: Johns Hopkins Center for Clinical Trials: 193-94.

[3] Fleming R, Demets DL (1996). Surrogate end points in clinical trials: are we being misled? *Ann Intern Med* 125: 605-13.

[4] Smigel K (1995). Women flock to ABMT for breast cancer without final proof. *J Natl Cancer Inst* 87: 952-55.

[5] Cutler CM, Udvarhelyi IS, Winkenwerder W (1994). Variations in insurance coverage for autologous bone marrow transplantation for breast cancer. *N Engl J Med* 331: 329-30.

[6] Weiss RB, Rifkin RM, et al. (2000). High-dose chemotherapy for high-risk primary breast cancer: an on-site review of the Bezwoda study. *Lancet* 355: 999-1003.

[7] McCarthy M (1996). Unproven breast-cancer therapy widely used in USA. *Lancet* 347: 1617.

[8] Triozzi PL (1994). Autologous bone marrow and peripheral blood progenitor transplant for breast cancer. *Lancet:* 344: 418-19.

[9] Gilyatt, P. (July 1995). Bone-marrow transplants. *Harvard Health Letter:* 3-5.

[10] Gottlieb S (1999). Bone marrow transplants do not help in breast cancer. *BMJ* 318: 1093.

[11] Bezwoda WR, Seymour L, Dansey RD (1995). High-dose chemotherapy with hematopoietic rescue as primary treatment for metastatic breast cancer: a randomized trial. *J Clin Oncol* 13: 2483-89.

[12] American Society for Clinical Oncology. High-dose chemotherapy with bone marrow transplant for breast cancer patients. http://www.asco.org/people/nr/html/genpr/m_0300bmtposition.htm, accessed on May 20, 2000.

[13] The Cardiac Arrhythmia Suppression Trial (CAST) Investigators (1989). Preliminary report: effect of encainide and flecainide on mortality in a randomized trial of arrhythmia suppression after myocardial infarction. *N Engl J Med* 321: 406-12.

[14] Moore TJ (1995). *Deadly medicine. Why tens of thousands of heart patients died in America's worst drug disaster.* New York: Simon & Schuster.

[15] Echt DS, Liebson PR, et al (1991). Mortality and morbidity in patients receiving encainide flecainide, or placebo. The Cardiac Arrhythmia Suppression Trial. *N Engl J Med* 324: 781-88.

[16] Fleming TR, Prentice RL, Pepe MS (1994). Surrogate and auxiliary endpoints in clinical trials, with potential applications in cancer and AIDS research. *Statistics Med* 13: 955-68.

[17] Crossen C (1994). *Tainted truth. The manipulation of fact in America.* New York: Simon & Schuster: 160-91.

[18] de Semir V (1996). What is newsworthy? *Lancet* 347: 1163-66.

[19] Simes RJ (1987). Confronting publication bias: a cohort design for meta-analysis. *Statistics Med* 6: 11-29.

[20] Egger M, Davey Smith G (1998). Meta-analysis: bias in location and selection of studies. *BMJ* 316: 61-66.

[21] Easterbrook PJ, Berlin J, et al. (1991). Publication bias in clinical research. *Lancet* 337: 867-72.

[22] Stern JM, Simes RJ (1997). Publication bias: evidence of delayed publication in a cohort study of clinical research projects. *BMJ* 315: 640-45.

[23] Ioannidis JPA (1998). Effect of the statistical significance of results on the time to completion and publication of randomized efficacy trials. *JAMA* 279: 281-86.

[24] Ravnskov U (1992). Cholesterol lowering trials in coronary heart disease: frequency of citation and outcome. *BMJ* 305: 15-19.

[25] Huston P, Moher D (1996). Redundancy, disaggregation, and the integrity of medical research. *Lancet* 347: 1024-26.

[26] Tramèr MR, Reynolds DJM, et al. (1997). Impact of covert duplicate publication on meta-analysis: a case study. *BMJ* 315: 635-40.

[27] Rennie D (1999). Fair conduct and fair reporting of clinical trials. *JAMA* 282: 1766-68.

[28] Horton R & Smith R (1999). Time to register randomized trials. *Lancet* 354: 1138-39.

[29] Yamey G (1999). Scientists who do not publish trial results are "unethical." *BMJ* 319: 939.

[30] Cochrane Collaboration Secretariat. http://hiru.mcmaster.ca/cochrane/resource.htm. Accessed January 9, 2000.

[31] Krimsky S, Rothenberg LS (1998). Financial interest and its disclosure in scientific publications. *JAMA* 280: 225-26.

[32] Holden C (2000). NEJM admits breaking its own tough rules. *Science* 287: 1573.

[33] Dickersin K, Min YL, Meinert CL (1992). Factors influencing publication of research results. Follow-up of applications submitted to two institutional review boards. *JAMA* 267: 374-78.

[34] Davidson RA (1986). Source of funding and outcome of clinical trials. *J Gen Intern Med* 1: 155-58.

[35] Rochon PA, Gurwitz JH, et al. (1994). A study of manufacturer-supported trials of nonsteroidal anti-inflammatory drugs in the treatment of arthritis. *Arch Intern Med* 154: 157-63.

[36] Sharp D (1998). A ghostly crew. *Lancet* 351: 1076.

[37] Begg C, Cho M, et al. (1996). Improving the quality of reporting of randomized controlled trials. The CONSORT statement. *JAMA* 276: 637-39.

[38] Schulz KF (1996). Randomised trials, human nature, and reporting guidelines. *Lancet* 348: 596-98.

[39] Shepherd J, Cobbe SM, et al. (1995). Prevention of coronary heart disease with pravastatin in men with hypercholesterolemia. West of Scotland Coronary Prevention Study Group. *N Engl J Med* 333: 1301-07.

[40] Hux JE, Naylor CD (1995). Communicating the benefits of chronic preventive therapy: does the format of efficacy data determine patients' acceptance of treatment? *Med Decis Making* 15: 152-57.

[41] Bucher HC, Weinbacher M, Gyr K (1994). Influence of method of reporting study results on decision of physicians to prescribe drugs to lower cholesterol concentration. *BMJ* 309: 761-64.

[42] Cranney M, Walley T (1996). Same information, different decisions: the influence of evidence on the management of hypertension in the elderly. *Br J Gen Pract* 46: 661-63.

[43] Naylor CD, Chen E, Strauss B (1992). Measured enthusiasm: does the method of reporting trial results alter perceptions of therapeutic effectiveness? *Ann Intern Med* 117: 916-21.

[44] Skolbekken JA (1998). Communicating the risk reduction achieved by cholesterol reducing drugs. *BMJ* 316: 1956-58.

[45] Greenhalgh T (1997). How to read a paper. Statistics for the non-statistician. II: "Significant" relations and their pitfalls. *BMJ* 315: 422-25.

[46] Egger M, Schneider M, Davey Smith G (1998).   Spurious precision? Meta-analysis of observational studies. *BMJ* 316: 140-45.

[47] Deyo RA, Psaty BM, et al. (1997).   The messenger under attack - intimidation of researchers by special-interest groups. *N Engl J Med* 336: 1176-80.

[48] Psaty BM, Heckbert SR, et al. (1995). The risk of myocardial infarction associated with antihypertensive drug therapies. *JAMA* 274: 620-25.

[49] Brennan TA (1994). Buying editorials. *N Engl J Med* 331: 673-75.

Chapter Five

Leaping Over the Species' Gap: The Substitution of Humans by Other Animals in Testing of Procedures and Substances

Andrew Thompson

The necessity and ethicality of subjecting other species to deprivation, suffering, and death to find out things which may benefit humans has been a cantankerous issue for a long time, certainly since the beginning of the twentieth century. However, the issue has never really been approached from the world view that this book proposes; namely that of environmentalism and social justice. From this perspective medical research is "a grace," something which is a boon to the extent we can afford it, rather than "a necessity." What is a necessity are those activities that promote life for all species, both now and in the future. Where in the priority list of medical research should research that demands the sacrificial use of other animals fall? This chapter critically examines the scientific case for research using other animals in light of current knowledge and alternatives. The next examines the moral case for such research.

Suppose we wanted to find out the effectiveness of ice cream as a motivator on children in India. What we would probably do would be to go to India and set up experiments where representative samples of Indian children would be randomized into two groups. One group would be told they would be rewarded with ice cream for doing certain tasks (and would indeed be given it after completion of each task) and the other group would be promised nothing. What we certainly would not do would be offer ice cream to adults in Canada or any other country that we happen to live in, even in India, and see how they react. And we would certainly not offer ice cream to monkeys or white mice, even white mice genetically altered to have similar taste buds to humans. These other options, especially the ones involving other animals, may well be less expensive and less cumbersome to arrange, but would be it considered ridiculous to use them. The results from

59

A. Thompson and N.J. Temple (eds.), Ethics, Medical Research, and Medicine, 59–73.
© 2001 *Kluwer Academic Publishers. Printed in the Netherlands.*

the animal experiments, in particular, could not be trusted to be relevant to any human group, much less that of children in India.

But when it comes to potentially hazardous effects, this approach which is likely to be misleading is, almost without exception, used first. Instead of directly trying out the effect of a drug, a surgical procedure, an insertion of genetically-altered material, or an environmental change on a sample of those for whom the drug, procedure, material, or change is intended, the intervention is first tried out on monkeys, mice, guinea pigs, or still other animals. In many experiments it is done to the extreme with some or all of the animals in order to find out both the point at which the intervention might be effective and the point at which it is fatal. Even the survivors may not be safe in that it may be deemed necessary to kill and autopsy them in order to more fully determine the effects of the intervention.

The result of such studies is that we know what happens to captive nonhuman animals under laboratory conditions. The results might not even carry over to the same species in their natural surroundings, much less to humans. There are two reasons why this is so: one is that individuals within any species differ, often dramatically, from each other because of differences in their environments, internal and external, and in their genes. Anyone who has had a pet knows that, as does anyone who has an allergy. Some people die because of a single sting from a bee while others are bee keepers. Some are dangerously allergic to penicillin; others are not, and so forth throughout the ever-growing list of allergic reactions. The same drugs, Ritalin and Zylert, which are used to stimulate adults, are also used as a means to quiet down hyperactive children. In fact, no drug has exactly the same reaction on any two people, which is why physicians ask that we inform them of any adverse reactions to drugs.

The second, much more fundamental reason, is that of evolution. According to fossil evidence, the predecessor of the human species became distinct from its closest relatives over two million years ago.[1] Thus the difference between it and that of any other animal species is truly profound. Two million years of evolution means that every organ in our bodies differs significantly from those of other species. It is said that there is only two percent difference between the DNA of chimpanzees and ours.[2] This sort of statement can be very misleading since it seems like such a small difference. However, it takes only a 0.1 percent difference in the human genome to account for, along with environmental factors, the vast array of individual differences among humans.[3] Current attempts to "humanize" other animals through genetic manipulation in order to overcome the massive, automatic reaction of our immune systems to transplantation of their organs or to make them more like us to test cancer drugs clearly demonstrates scientists' awareness of the inadequacies of other animals as substitutes for humans in determining whole body functioning.

Researchers also reveal this awareness by virtue of the fact that they usually do not claim to have discovered anything of more than "initially promising" value in experiments on other animals until they have repeated the experiments on one or two other species and obtained consistent results. If this consistency indicates that the product, procedure, or environmental change is both useful and reasonably safe, they then proceed to experiment on humans. In many cases, they are required by regulatory agencies to use nonhumans first. The danger is that too much faith will be placed in the experimental results using other species and the investigators will do a less than thorough job sampling the broad spectrum of humans, ranging across sexes, ages, physical states, and environmental situations.

In reality, it is almost a sure thing that this testing is inadequate. For instance, it is estimated that it would require 30,000 human subjects to detect an adverse drug reaction that would affect one or more of 10,000 people. Yet only 1,500 are normally required to be tested by clinical trials to get approval for marketing.[4]

This problem is much more than of mere theoretical importance. Unanticipated, adverse reactions to prescribed drugs in prescribed amounts are among the leading causes of death in hospitals, the setting in which both the available expertise and the control over prescriptions would be assumed to be maximum. One can only wonder how many deaths are caused by prescriptions given outside of hospitals. Currently, it is impossible to find this out since such data are not likely to be systematically recorded, or made easily accessible. In addition, hospitals are reluctant to collect and release such information.[5] These adverse side effects are unanticipated, in part, because the laboratory animals did not show them. They are also unanticipated because, in many cases, a combination of drugs is prescribed, and this combination has <u>never</u> been tested on any animal, humans included. In fact, to adequately test all the various drug combinations that may be prescribed is currently an impossible task, since there are so many drugs, and more are constantly being approved for distribution. This makes for a dangerous situation. Given the vast array of drugs, individual differences in reactions, differences in the environments in which people live, and other confounding variables, physicians cannot be truly competent in the prescription of many, and probably most, of the drugs at their disposal.

Perhaps the most publicized example of inadequate testing of the relevant species was that of thalidomide. This widely used sedative was discovered to cause fetal abnormalities if taken in the first three months of pregnancy. Eight thousand children in 46 countries were born with malformations.[6] Yet this drug had passed the usual animal tests in Europe and was prescribed in a number of countries. After the pharmaceutical company finally admitted to having produced a crippling drug and did some further research, it found an animal that the drug did have adverse effects upon -- the New Zealand white rabbit. The reaction of critics was predictable. More animals of more species should have been used, especially pregnant animals.[7] Thalidomide ended up being tested on approximately 10 strains of rats, 15 of mice, 11 breeds of rabbits, two of dogs, three strains of hamsters, eight species of primates, and other varied species such as cats, armadillos, guinea pigs, swine, and ferrets -- with varying results. From them, one could not be sure which would be true also of humans. Testing a wider sample of humans, one which included fully informed pregnant women, would have exposed the problem much sooner and in a definitive manner. Several women would have had malformed children (if they were not identified before the birth and aborted), but certainly not 8000. If one considers the justification for the testing in the first place, it might not have been done at all. There was surely no compelling need for still another sedative on the market and even less need for giving it to pregnant women.[8]

The industry has taken another direction, however; they do more testing of pregnant animals. They have also found other possible uses for thalidomide but the question of how to be sure that pregnant women won't take it has not been fully answered.[6,9]

Thalidomide is far from being an exceptional example: other less well-publicized "miscalculations" abound. A Scientific American article lists four of them; all approved by the FDA for marketing.[10] Milrinone, a heart drug, increased survival of rats with artificially induced heart failure but was found to lead to a 30 percent increase in mortality in humans. Fialuridine, an antiviral drug, caused lived failure in seven of 15 patients, five of whom subsequently died and the other two required liver transplantations. Zomepirac sodium, a popular painkiller in the 1980s, was withdrawn from the market after it was implicated in 14 deaths and hundreds of life-threatening allergic reactions. The antidepressant nomifensive was withdrawn when it was found to cause sometimes fatal liver toxicity and anemia in humans. Altogether, an FDA review of 198 drugs released between 1976 and 1985 found that 52 percent of them posed serious risks to those who took them, risks that led to their relabeling or withdrawal from the market. With any less politically powerful industry this would have led to sharp curtailment of its activities. This in not a matter of science, but of misuse of power.

The unanticipated consequences suffered by humans who were prescribed these drugs were often serious or fatal but we should not overlook the predictable consequences on the animals used to determine the safety of the drugs. A standard test for such determination is the LD50 Test. It is so named because it determines what amount of a substance is fatal to 50 percent of a group of animals within 14 days. The researchers then kill the survivors and perform autopsies on them to determine the effects of poisoning. They do not relieve the misery the animals experience before dying since this might affect the results.[11,12]

It is often mandatory to extensively experiment on animals before experiments on humans.[13] The USA is particularly stringent in this area. Those substances considered to be potentially acutely toxic must be tested on three or four species: those of "subacute toxicity" require two species for three months or two species for six months. Chronic toxicity requires 12 months of testing on two strains of rats and 12 months on two breeds of dogs; and substances thought to be potentially cancer-causing must be tested for two years on rats and 18 months on mice.[14] Canada, on the other hand, requires the use of nonhuman species "only if the researcher's best efforts to find an alternative have failed" and "expert opinion must attest to the potential value of studies with animals."[15]

The shortcomings of the American position were recently made evident in a comment in *Time Magazine*.[16] In an experiment under the auspices of Amvac Chemical, small doses of a pesticide used to kill caterpillars were fed to human volunteers in England to investigate human tolerance to it. The Environmental Protection Agency of the USA (of all agencies!) refused to accept the study results and asked for animal tests instead. Somewhere alone the line common sense has been abandoned and indirect, prone-to-error methodology has replaced direct, trustworthy methodology.

These shortcomings are also quite evident simply by looking at other evidence for the lack of correlation between the effects of tests on laboratory animals and the effects of the same substances on human beings. The Medical Research Modernization Committee[17] has reviewed over 150 studies using such lab tests. A few examples of what they found will have to suffice here. One review reported that substances that cause cancer were found to not even carry over, for the most part, between different rodent species. On the other hand, substances known to cause cancer in humans may not do so in other animals. In one series that followed the standard National Cancer Institute protocol, only seven of 19 human carcinogens were found to also cause cancer in other animals. According to another study, stroke-reducing compounds fared even worse: zero of 25 compounds found to reduce stroke in nonhumans did so in humans. A review of four prevalent neurological diseases, including Alzheimer's, found that animal studies contributed little to nothing to the understanding or treatment of the illnesses.

The basic argument for the use of other animals in research that would be hazardous or simply unpalatable to humans is that one level of research requires the use of live animals - research that has reached the point where one needs to determine how the body functions as an integrated whole. Drugs that are taken orally, for example, may be metabolized into more active, even toxic, substances in one organ before acting on other organs. One cannot replicate fully the complexity of behavioral and physiological reactions and interactions of live organisms.

However, as we have seen, experimentation on whole, live, nonhuman animals does not tell us much about what will happen to humans since the organs of other animals differ significantly from ours, with the result that any interactions among them will also differ in unknown ways. The interactions may also vary due to the broad range of circumstances that exist outside of the experimental situation. Equally important, these differences are almost bound to increase greatly over time so that it would be foolish to predict what would happen five, ten, or fifteen years later. Many effects also only reveal themselves under certain conditions, such as occurs when organs, damaged by age, are no longer able to compensate for the damage caused by earlier treatment. The only way to determine these effects is to conduct long-term research on humans, not 12-month studies on rats. Scientists show their awareness of this fact in their use of mathematical models that they have developed from comparing data from experiments on other animals to those on humans. These models are then used to project the data from experiments on other animals unto humans, thus reducing the number of experimental animal subjects. Such models are limited to immediate reactions, not long-term ones.[18] Also, all such mathematical models must be tested periodically, which then requires more tests on laboratory animals.

The scientists and lab workers who inflict harm on other animals as part of the process of developing cosmetics and household products can be assumed to do so, to a large part, because they believe such research to be necessary to protect humans and that the products that result are beneficial to many people. Even those who are not so sure about the protective and useful value of the research are not likely to refuse to engage in such hurtful and deadly practices because to do so would likely cost them their jobs. Other motives come into larger play in medical research, especially research that attempts to prove or disprove a new theory or explore a new field. Let us provide a few examples of such research that helped establish the careers and the reputations of particular researchers, starting with one from the field of psychology.

Harry Harlow became famous partially because of experiments his research group conducted on baby monkeys in an attempt to find out how human infants might respond to various kinds of mistreatment.[11,19] Among other things, Harlow decided to study the psychological state of depression in human infants by inducing it in infant monkeys. This proved to be tougher than anticipated. First, the infant monkeys were forcibly separated from their mothers and given cloth-covered, wire-framed surrogates which they learned to cling to. Since that by itself did not induce depression, the monkeys were progressively subjected to emission of high-pressured air from the surrogates, rocking severe enough to rattle the infant monkeys' teeth and heads, ejection by the springing out of the embedded wire frame, and finally ejection by sharp brass spikes emerging from their surrogate mothers. None of these produced the desired results.

"Depression" was finally achieved by placing the baby monkeys in a vertical chamber with stainless steel sides sloping inwards to form a rounded bottom, where they stayed for up to 45 days. After a while they remained huddled in a corner of the chamber.

Harlow's experiments were widely publicized in the professional literature as having discovered basic truths about the care of children. I remember reading descriptions of some of the milder experiments in texts for basic and advanced psychology courses during the late 1950s and early 1960s. Even at that time I had some question as to how much resemblance taking monkeys away from their mothers and giving them cloth-covered wire frames had to any human infant situations. After all, we already knew how useful teddy bears are in pacifying children. Application to care of monkeys was even more inconceivable. I was probably not alone in my doubts but heard only praise for these oft-quoted experiments from colleagues and professors. However, things may be changing. A commentary some years later stated: "It is easy to understand why many clinicians and investigators have been extremely skeptical of alleged animal models of depression."[19]

Hans Selye gained fame based on his research and writings on stress. He experimented on rats to determine the biological mechanisms activated by various kinds of stress. The rats were surgically injured, starved for 48 hours or more, exposed to cold or to restraints for prolonged periods, and given toxic doses of various chemicals and drugs. Some were made quadriplegic. The internal effects included gastrointestinal ulcers, atrophy of ovaries, cardiac hypertrophy, appendicitis, and death.[11,19] How relevant this was or how much this added to our knowledge of what happens to people in dire circumstances, much less what we can do for them, remains a matter of speculation.

Another series of studies that was intended to shed light on human psychological functioning was carried out at the University of Western Michigan.[11] It subjected rats to electric shocks, intense enough in some cases to cause paralysis and even death. In one such study a pair of rats received 15,000 shocks in 7.5 hours; in another, five rats were shocked every day for 80 days, with the result that they engaged in vicious fights in which they suffered severe cuts and bruises.

The chief investigator re-evaluated his work 16 years later in these terms:

> *Initially my research was prompted by the desire to understand and help solve the problem of human aggression but I later discovered that the results of my work did not seem to justify its continuance. Instead, I began to wonder if perhaps financial rewards, professional prestige, the opportunity to travel etc., were the maintaining factors, and if we of the scientific community (supported by our bureaucratic and legislative system) were actually a part of the problem"* (p. 102 of footnote 11).

Both this research and the team of researchers under Harlow's tutelage were caught up in the Zeitgeist of the time: the belief that all animals, including humans, respond to common laws of nature and thus share common feelings of depression and aggression as a result of painful experiences and frustration. Since then we have learned much more about how other animals live from studying them in their natural environments. We now realize that in an artificial environment, both their individual and their group interactive behavior changes greatly, and, in any case, is quite distinctive from that of humans. Such environmental studies may teach us not to make such simplistic leaps of faith across the species gap.

Despite these lessons, the tendency to make the species leap to study newly "discovered" (i.e., hypothesized) psychological states such as "learned helplessness" still exists. The problem is, from the experimenter's point of view, that it would be "inhuman" and, in any case, probably not allowed to try to induce such a state in humans for scientific purposes. Thus, the temptation is to do it on laboratory animals, with the hope that one can get something that looks like learned helplessness and write up the results for publication. Being that it is a new, interesting theory, the chances are good the paper will see publication. And if published, then it is easier to get funding for follow up studies, still on nonhumans, of course, because of the difficulties of studying humans. One publication leads to another, with each set of authors supporting each other in this credential-gaining, growing field. The fact that the knowledge gained is about other animals in laboratory conditions and not humans in real-life situations is worrisome, and always mentioned, but this does not stop the rewards from coming in.

There is a range of alternatives to research on substitute animals and we will look at these a little later, but one we will mention now is that of population (epidemiological) studies on people. For example, instead of harmfully treating baby monkeys to find out what might make human infants depressed, one could search for such infants and determine what circumstances are common in their lives which might account for their depression. Are most of them undernourished? Neglected? Mistreated in some other way? Scientists find such studies inadequate in that they cannot control what happened to the individuals being studied and thus determine with any certainty the direct effects of environmental changes. Additionally, epidemiological studies require different skills, non-laboratory skills, skills which many researchers do not have. Finally, the generalization of the results are less sure, albeit vastly more relevant, and their interpretation often easily challenged, thus requiring replication to gain wider acceptance. This can make publications more problematic, and without publications one cannot advance in many scientific careers.

For the reasons described above a whole industry has built up that specializes in animal research. Let us briefly look at the size of the industry and the rules that regulate it. Doing so will help us further understand why it is resistant to questioning one of its basic assumptions, the assumption that other animals are adequate substitutes in doing research on interventions intended for humans.

HOW LARGE IS THIS ANIMAL-FOR-HUMAN RESEARCH INDUSTRY?

It is difficult to determine exactly how many animals are used as substitutes for humans in research projects, because, for one thing, it is such a huge enterprise with a wide variety of facilities in a variety of institutions under a number of different private and public auspices. Also, due to reluctance to provide "ammunition" to animal rights and animal welfare groups and fear of the public reaction that may ensue, institutions do not normally volunteer to release data showing how many animals of what kind they use in their research. Some European countries do, however, collect systematic data on animal pain and distress. According to a 1990 report of research in the Netherlands[20], 53 percent of animals used in research suffered minor discomfort, 23 percent moderate, and 24 percent severe. Basel, Switzerland, hosts several scientific institutions, two of which are international pharmaceutical giants, Novartis and Hoffman-Roche. The Basel institutions report to the government how many animals they use in their research and place these numbers in categories of distress they have to undergo: benign, mild, medium, and severe. Almost one third of the 288,564 animals in 1998 were in the medium to severe categories.

However, these records and the facilities are not open to members of the general public.[21,22] If they were so, these numbers may very well be distributed differently, at least according to what sociologist Mary Phillips observed was true of researchers in the USA.[17] Nonhuman species were subjected to toxicity tests, cancer-inducing procedures, major surgery operations, and other painful protocols. Yet, in annual reports to the federal authorities, there was no acknowledgement that any animals experienced unrelieved pain or distress, being that the researchers defined pain to refer only to the acute pain of surgery on conscious animals.

In 1997, the United Kingdom authorities reported that about 2.66 million "scientific procedures" were carried out in that country.[23] The number of animals having a genetic defect increased by 10 percent and those who were genetically modified by 27 percent, which may account for the increase in animals involved over the previous year.

The United States Department of Agriculture's 1998 report lists 1.2 million animals of which about 760,000 were rabbits, hamsters, and guinea pigs with most of the rest consisting of dogs, primates, and cats.[24] In addition, 23 million rats, mice, and birds were used in 1999 in the nation's laboratories. They are listed separately since they, although warm-blooded, are not protected under the Animal Welfare Act which prescribes the temperature, ventilation, and space in which animals are to be kept.[25]

The portion used for education purposes has been estimated at only one percent but this is not insignificant in terms of teaching students attitudes towards animals. An educator at Georgetown University in Washington DC explained why they decided to close down their vivarium in these words[26]:

> *For many years, members of our faculty and our undergraduates considered the ethical basis upon which persons would maintain sentient and complex animals in confinement and for purposes that did not appear to bear upon any significant human concern. In time, the traditional defenses seemed to most to be self-serving and entirely unconvincing, not to mention at variance with any number of ethical principles carefully examined in any number of undergraduate courses in philosophy.*

According to Michael Fox[19] in his book defending animal research, *The Case for Animal Experimentation,* about 40 percent of all animals are used for scientific biomedical and behavioral research, 26 percent for drug development, and 20 percent for toxicity testing. What happens to the other 14 percent is not clear but some of that is probably for military research. Actually, these figures seem to be gross underestimates since Bernard Rollin, a philosopher who has specialized in the ethics of using animals for research, claims that the US Department of Defense "is the largest consumer of laboratory animals in the world" (p. 167 of footnote 12).

This is not without financial benefit to the institutions that support this research. Large medical centers, for example, annually receive tens of millions of dollars in direct grants for medical research and tens of millions more for supposedly related overhead costs.[17]

ANIMAL CARE REGULATIONS -- WHAT ROLE DO THEY PLAY?

Because of the lobbying by animal protectionists, federal legislation has been passed in the USA that provides standards for the protection and welfare of some of the animals used for medical research.[27,28] It may be thought that these regulations truly prevent exploitation of animals. This is highly questionable. First of all, the rules are enforced by oversight committees consisting of five members who are appointed by the chief executive officer of the institution in which the research takes place. Thus, these committees can be expected to be weighted to represent the institution's interests. Such committees are supposed to allow for participation by citizen groups and other interested parties and each institutional committee is supposed to have at least one member that represents the community. However, the likelihood that an animal rightists would be chosen is slim. It can be easily argued that, given only one public representative, it would be better to choose someone more representative of the public and less apt to be obstructive to the work of the committee.

Many who are committed to such research find such restrictions to be an unnecessary interference and argue that scientists can be trusted to police themselves.[29] Yet how strict is the scientific oversight at the crucial stage, the approval of the proposal? The National Institute of Health policy only requires that the sections that relate to the care and use of animals be available to members of Institutional Animal Care and Use Committees. There is no explicit requirement that the sections that describe what is to be done, and why, are to be made available. Without the whole proposal, its basic scientific merit cannot be determined, and without such a review, it is not possible to decide whether the potential benefits of the research justifies the known harm to the animals.[30] But even a full review would be one conducted by an institutional committee in which the members may well be colleagues of the investigators, thus introducing an uncritical bias in favor of the proposal.

The probable real effect of these regulations is some improvement of the confinement conditions of some animals and elimination or scaling down of some research projects because of the additional effort and expense that has to be done to get them approved.

WHAT ARE THE ALTERNATIVES?

A number of things are clear at this point:

1) the effort to protect humans from pain, suffering, and even death from experimental procedures and products has led to a lot of pain, suffering, and death of other species;

2) the results of this experimentation on other species are known not to be trustworthy and could not be expected to be, given the facts of individual and evolutionary differences within and between species; hence, further experimentation is required on humans themselves;

3) that this further experimentation has often proven inadequate – humans are still all too likely to suffer adverse consequences, including death, from the "approved" products and procedures; and

4) that an industry has built up around this system of experimentation, an industry that rewards those who participate in it in a number of ways, starting with basic employment for many up to fame and fortune for a few.

Hence, any other approach will meet with resistance, very likely, a great deal of resistance. We shall go into this latter point at length in the next chapter. For now, let us look at the alternatives that do exist.

Epidemiology - as mentioned before this is the examination of statistical data on the incidence of disease in various populations. For example, how many coal miners die of lung diseases as opposed to people in general? And what characterizes those miners who contract such diseases from those who do not?

Molecular Epidemiology - an emerging science that relates epidemiological data on disease incidence to genetic, metabolic, and biochemical factors.

In vitro (test tube) testing of substances on various cultures or tissues. For example, trying out a new drug on a cancer cell culture. Or testing the effects of insertion of a certain substance on tissue from an aborted fetus. These methodologies have the additional advantage of being incredibly efficient. Screening of 100 *in vitro* human cancer cell lines, for example, would largely replace the screening done from the mid-1950s to the mid-1980s of 400,000 possible anticancer agents on nonhuman subjects.

Human fetal tissue is considered by leading medical ethical committees as deserving higher moral concern than live laboratory animals; so approval of such experimentation is often hard to obtain.[31,32,33]

Use of human cadavers in medical training, as medical students do in various countries, in conjunction with artificial models, diagrams, and films. Also, use of the human placenta for training in microvascular surgery.

Computer programs using mathematical models can predict the toxicity of drugs or project the effects of substances or procedures on various organs.

High-performance liquid chromatography can measure hormone and antihumor antibiotic levels; positron emission tomography can provide images of the human brain in action.

Mass spectrometry and gas spectrometry can aid in analysis of human and animal blood, and saturation analysis.

Radio-immunoassy can measure hormone concentration in tissues.

Given all the various alternatives to experimenting on other animals and the predictive inaccuracy of tests on them, we might well ask if we need to experiment on them at all. Why not limit medical research to that which involves these alternatives? We could expand direct experimentation on humans after use of the alternatives. This would be done in a very cautious manner involving fully voluntary and informed, subjects. Such safeguards would insure that the case for the research is truly a strong one, not one involving development of still another "me too" product or a product or procedure which promises only minimal improvement, or improvement limited to only those few who can afford it.

References

[1] Associated Press (March 23, 2000). Did humans evolve from knuckle-walkers? *Register-Guard*, Eugene, OR: 5A

[2] Jameton A (1996). Human activity and environmental ethics. In: Thomasma DC, Kushner T, eds. *Birth to death: science and bioethics.* Cambridge, England: Cambridge University Press: 357-67.

[3] Bonn D (1999). International consortium SN(I)Ps away at individuality. *Lancet* 353: 1684.

[4] Pirmohamed M, Breckenbridge AM, et al. (1998). Adverse drug reactions. *BMJ* 316: 1295-98.

[5] Lazarou J, Pomeranz BH, Corey PN (1998). Incidence of adverse drug reactions in hospitalized patients. *JAMA* 279: 1200-05.

[6] A cautious comeback for thalidomide (February 4, 1998). *Harvard Health Letter*: 4.

[7] Kaley H (November, 1990). Animal tests and thalidomide. *American Psychological Association Monitor*: 2.

[8] Bowd AD (February, 1991). How much is enough? *American Psychological Association Monitor*: 3.

[9] Stephenson J (1999). FDA weighs communicating drug-related risks to patients. *JAMA* 282: 515.

[10] Barnard ND, Kaufman SR (February, 1997). Animal research is wasteful and misleading. *Scientific American*: 80-82. Accessed through http://www.mrmed.org/critcv.html

[11] Sharpe R (1988). *The cruel deception: the use of animals in medical research.* Wellingborough, Northhamptonshire, England: Thorsons Publishers.

[12] Rollin BE (1990). *The unheeded cry: animal consciousness, animal pain, and science.* Oxford: Oxford University Press.

[13] Weidmann H (June 18,1998). Sittliche Verpflichtung des Forschers. *Basler Zeitung,* Switzerland: 31

[14] Sherman M, Strauss S (1996). A capsuled history of drug law in the U.S. In: Strauss S, ed. *Strauss's Federal Drug Laws and Examination Review* (4th Ed). Lancaster, Pennsylvania: Technomic Publishing Company: 171-86.

[15] Brody BA (1998). *The ethics of biomedical research: an international perspective.* New York: Oxford University Press: 338.

[16] If it kills caterpillars, what about people? (August 10, 1998). *Time*: 10.

[17] Cohen MJ, Kaufman SR, et al. (1998). A critical look at animal experimentation. *Medical Research Modernization Committee.* Accessed February 4, 2000, at http//www.mrmcmed.org/critcv.html.

[18] Dell D (September, 1999). Retired pharmaceutical company analytical chemist and laboratory administrator. Personal communication noted when he read the chapter.

[19] Fox MA (1986). *The case for animal experimentation.* Berkley: University of California Press: 215.

[20] Loew FM (1996). Animals in research. In: Thomasma DC, Kushner T, eds. *Birth to death: science and bioethics.* Cambridge, England: Cambridge University Press: 301-12.

[21] Die Zahl der Teirversuche hat sich stabilisiert (July 22, 1999). *Basler Zeitung,* Switzerland: 27.

[22] Tausz-Weber B (August 18, 1997). Alle Tierversuche verbieten. *Basler Zeitung,* Switzerland: 28.

[23] Berger A (1999). Animal tests rise in Great Britain. *BMJ* 319: 402.

[24] Report of the Secretary of Agriculture. *Animal welfare report,* 1998. Washington, DC: USDA.

[25] New York Times (October 15, 2000). Researchers win delay of rules. *Register Guard,* Eugene, OR: 4A.

[26] Robinson DN (November, 1990). Comment on animal research labs. *American Psychologist*: 1269.

[27] Rowan AN (May-June, 1990). Section IV: Ethical review and the Animal Care and Use Committee. Hastings Center Report: 19-24.

[28] Public Health Service (September, 1986). *Public Health Service Policy on Humane Care and Use of Laboratory Animals.* Washington, DC.

[29] Weissmann G (1979). Science for science's sake. In: Bruce Bohle, ed. *Human life: controversies and concerns.* New York: Pantheon Books: 26-33.

[30] Finsen L (1989). Institutional Animal Care and Use Committees: a new set of clothes for the emperor? In: Beauchamp TL, Walters L, eds. *Contemporary issues in bioethics.* Belmont, CA: Wadsworth Publishing Company: 484-89.

[31] Culliton BJ (December 23, 1988). Panel backs fetal tissue research. *Science*: 1625-26.

[32] Engelhardt HT (1986). *The foundations of bioethics*. New York: Oxford University Press.
[33] Coutts MC (March, 1993). Fetal tissue research. *Kennedy Institute of Ethics Journal*: 81-101.

Chapter Six

The Moral Justification for Substituting Other Animals in Medical Research
Andrew Thompson

A biomedical research establishment without animals would be like an army without infantry, and it may as well be admitted that animals are sometimes the cannon fodder in the battle against disease. Thomas Malone[1]

If animals are sufficiently similar to humans to be good models, what right do we have to do to them what we would not do to humans? Bernard Rollin[2]

Depriving humans (and animals) of advances in medicine that result from research on animals is inhumane and fundamentally unethical. Loeb et al.[3]

A thing is right when it tends to preserve the integrity, stability, and beauty of the biotic community. It is wrong when it tends otherwise. Aldo Leopold[4]

The relationship between the animal research industry and those who oppose such use of other animals is not a very gentlemanly one: rather it is one of trying to ignore the bothersome pest on one side and seeking an audience on the other. Franklin M. Loew[5], dean of the College of Veterinary Medicine at Cornell University has described it in these terms: "The research establishment has shown little interest in debating the technical merits of animal research with their critics for fear it may give the critics what is perceived to be undeserved legitimacy." The establishment apparently extends to the National Institute of Health in that it joins many research advocacy organizations in rejecting using the term "alternative," preferring "adjunct" and "complimentary methods." Loew[5] adds that "alternative" is seen "as a Trojan Horse planted by the animal protection movement that will lead to great harm for medical research if allowed to gain a foothold."

75

A. Thompson and N.J. Temple (eds.), Ethics, Medical Research, and Medicine, 75–94.
© 2001 Kluwer Academic Publishers. Printed in the Netherlands.

Loew[5] further notes how unequal the two sides are in terms of political strength. The early successes of the animal protectionists were in the 1970s and 1980s when they enjoyed a good press. But then the tide turned as scientific organizations and pressure groups formed to defend animal research and mobilized the available resources: superior funding, sophisticated public relations skills, excellent contacts with the media, and high profile, respected spokespersons. "Given the skills and contacts available to the research and testing community, it could be considered something of a surprise that the animal protection community can point to any positive stories in the past few years, let alone still to be holding their own." They have not held their own in Congress, however. Loew[5] makes the point that the medical lobby managed to get legislation introduced and signed into law that singled out and made theft and destruction of a research facility a federal crime and subject to the jurisdiction of the FBI.

Given this inequality of power the interaction between medical researchers and animal protectionists can be compared to a public debate in which the party that enjoys the commanding position doesn't show up. There is a greater risk that it would lose public support than there is that it would gain any, whereas the reverse is true for the party which has, at the moment, little public support. This party is then stuck with the task of somehow reaching the public in other ways if it wants a fair and full hearing. This is not easy, and sometimes groups within the party in the inferior position resort to various kinds of protests, including illegal acts, as a means of getting media attention to their cause, and also perhaps, as a way of venting their frustration. In view of the political imbalance in presentation of issues, this chapter provides a comprehensive presentation of the ethical issues involved in the substitution of other animals for humans in medical research.

The "White Paper on Animal Research" serves as an entry into the research establishment's supporting arguments. This paper was commissioned by the American Medical Association and an condensation of it was published in 1989 in *JAMA*, its official journal. The introductory abstract reads: "The American Medical Association has long been a defender of humane research that employs animals, and it is very concerned about the efforts of animal rights and welfare groups to interfere with research[3]." "Defender of," "interfere with," and the reference to "animals" as if humans are not also animals is not the sort of language consistent with attempting to approach the issue with an open mind.

The paper goes on by listing a number of medical advances that are credited to research on laboratory animals. It then takes a moral stance: "From this perspective, depriving humans (and animals) of advances in medicine that result from research with animals is inhumane and fundamentally unethical." The "perspective" is that of the immorality of <u>not</u> using other animals as human substitutes.

The same dogmatic tone is expressed by McCloskey[6] in a book on medical ethics:

> *Most accounts of the ethics of human experimentation insist, rightly, that experiments on human beings are morally desirable only if embarked upon after all the relevant preliminary animal experiments have been carried out. To forbid experiments on animals but to permit experimentation on human conscripts and/or human volunteers who are made necessary because animal experimentation is outlawed is morally outrageous.*

He does not provide any reasons why it is morally outrageous in this article, perhaps assuming that they are obvious to his readers.

The previous chapter questioned one of the basic premises of those who defend using other animals as substitutes for humans. It is that, despite the gap between species caused by millions of years of evolution, other animals are similar enough to humans that valuable information for humans can be found out by experimenting on them. This chapter continues by critically examining the beliefs and arguments, often implicit, that constitute the case for the proponents of research on other animals in the hope of human benefit.

Let us start with one of the other central underlying beliefs that underlie this research and which the *JAMA* article presents as a fact. It is that an essential component of most, of all medical advances in the past decades has been the use of other animals as substitutes for humans in research. That this is a belief, and not necessarily a fact, becomes clear when we realize that it is impossible to know whether what has been discovered could not have been discovered by other means. Some useful discoveries may never have been made without experimentation on other animals, but it is also possible that if other means had been used instead, ones not involving laboratory animals, that other useful discoveries would have been made that were not made. We just don't know what would have happened because alternative means for exploring the same issues have been very limited in scope, with few, if any, attempts to directly compare the two approaches. Nevertheless, the bulk of research money is dedicated to research which sacrifices other animals in the preliminary stages, and, indeed, it is "essential" to do so because of legal stipulations in several countries.

Let us now look at the more clearly ethical, rather than scientific justifications that are offered in support of research on laboratory animals. It is unquestionable that it would be "imprudent" to use humans in many of the experiments that are done on other animals but is it really "moral" to use other animals instead? We will start with a brief overview of the general philosophical positions and then look at specific arguments.

Baruch Brody[7] divided the philosophical positions into five kinds. Descartes was the first to provide a definitive, comprehensive position. He maintained that the welfare of other animals was not really of consideration, "either because animals are incapable of feeling pain and suffering losses or because humans are morally entitled to disregard any animal pain or losses."

The second, advanced first by Henry Salt and later by Tom Regan, considers other animals, at least mammals, to also have their own, individual, inner life, including a sense of their future and sense of identity over time. Hence, they are entitled to the same rights as humans and should not be subjected to any research that harms them or risks harming them, unless it benefits the animal subjects themselves or is a case of "extreme necessity."[8]

The other three positions are between these two. The "human priority" position puts human interests above those of other animals but would have us minimize the suffering and losses of these animals to the extent possible without seriously interfering with the research. The "balancing position" grants humans the most consideration but says that, in cases of sufficient importance, the interests of other animals can take precedence. The "equal consideration" position, attributed to Peter Singer, grants equal consideration to humans and other animals. However, other animals are less sensitive to some losses and suffer less than humans in some experiments so they can be substituted for humans in such research. The gains for humans must be sufficient to outweigh the suffering and losses the substitute animals experience.

What is missing from all of these positions is an environmental, social-justice perspective, the one adopted by this book and presented in Chapter One. This perspective does not automatically or implicitly grant special considerations to the human species as a whole and certainly not to a minority of presently living, well-off individuals at the expense of other humans and other animals, current and future. The most protective position described above, that of Salt-Regan, shows little sensitivity to freedom-robbing experimentation on other animals and provides for exceptions to the prohibition of harm-causing experimentation in cases of extreme emergency -- for humans, thus clearly giving the nod to humans in terms of protection.

The arguments that immediately follow are those that are commonly expressed by researchers who conduct such experiments, and thus, in some ways and to some people, carry more weight than the theoretical positions sketched above.

One argument is that we are really doing the animals a favor by using them. The starting point for this argument is that the vast majority of the animals used are bred solely for research and therefore owe their lives to the presence of such research.[9] The assumption underlying this argument is that life, in and of itself, regardless of its quality, is of positive value. We can expose the barrenness of this argument very quickly: all we have to do is to apply it to humans. Under this assumption, conceiving and raising extra children for the sole purpose of using them in life-restricting, potentially harmful medical research would be not only a permitted but a valued activity. But when we talk about life itself being a boon, we always impart a minimum level of quality.

This consideration also applies to an allied argument; namely, that life in medical breeding stations and laboratories may be as good as, if not better than, life in the wild, given that the lab animals are assured of adequate food and warmth and are protected from predators.[10] What is ignored is that breeding and raising animals for generations in artificial surroundings does not make such surroundings the habitats for which their genes have prepared them. Nor does separating them from their parents and their natural groupings and confining them in artificial boundaries and in equipment-dominated, rectangular surroundings, begin to compare to the richness, complexity, and choice present in a natural, healthy habitat.

A "pure science" argument is that such research is justified simply on the basis of human curiosity.[9] Again, the hidden assumption is exposed by applying such reasoning to experimentation on humans. Curiosity does not carry much ethical weight when it comes to torturing, maiming, and killing humans for the sake of medical research, even though such research may satisfy the curiosity of the experimenters. In fact, the major international guidelines -- the Nuremburg Code, the Declaration of Helsinki, and the Belmont Report -- require much more than scientific curiosity as a justification for any research hazardous to human subjects.[11]

It is difficult to understand this apparent indifference shown by those who make the above arguments to the well-being – emotional, psychological and physical – of laboratory animals. Steven Kaufman,[12] co-chair of the Modern Research Modernization Committee, an antivivisectionist group, says that some researchers "openly state that they care more about humans than non humans." The implication is that this caring has argumentative weight. Certainly, we all are free to care for whom we will, but this does not justify inflicting harm on others, human or nonhuman. Caring only justifies doing something special for others. It does not justify harming those you don't care about.

Another argument is that such research sometimes also helps animals. It is claimed that vaccines and other treatments designed for

human use and developed with the help of animal surrogates have saved the lives of millions of animals. It is even speculated that the knowledge gained from inducing fear in primates in laboratory conditions can be used to help conservation programs reintroduce zoo-bred primates and other animals back into wilderness preserves.[3,13]

It may well be that some vaccines that have been developed for use by humans have also been successful against infectious animal diseases, particularly those which are spread in domesticated animals that are kept in confined spaces. That is, there is a sort of incidental, "trickle down" effect. But, if we were really concerned with fighting animal diseases, we would probably have arrived at these vaccines much quicker by doing the research for their benefit in the first place. There would be no need to induce the disease in lab animals, try out various substances on them, and then try them out on us, and then try them out on animals in their natural environments. This way the errors involved in inducing diseases in laboratory animals who are stressed by their artificial environments would be eliminated. Such reactions are far less trustworthy, less predictable of what would happen, even to their own species living in natural conditions.

The claim that inducing fear in primates in laboratories will somehow tell us how to reduce that fear in animals who are to be returned to the wild is also hard to take seriously. Those actually engaged in such restorative work have no doubt, by trial and error and clinical observation, learned far more of value in this line than from any laboratory-induced fear in animals.

A reverse argument is that some treatments that are developed for animals have been found to work on humans as well. If so, that is all for the good. This doesn't demonstrate that it is a good way to develop treatments for humans, however. We would never think of doing so. But once the treatment works on one species it is possible that it might work on another. But it doesn't prove that this is the best was to go about finding out what would work on the other. Think of the uproar if it were suggested that we find out what works on other animals by first using humans as guinea pigs. It would be declared unethical and unscientific in no time flat.

Humane treatment of animals in laboratories reduces their misery to an acceptable level. This argument is often implied rather than stated explicitly but seems to be a key argument of proponents of research on laboratory animals. It is claimed that many of the research animals are subject to mild, even benign, treatment. Reducing intervention to a benign level refers primarily to reducing or eliminating any intervention-associated pain by means of anesthetics. This may satisfy some animal protectionists that view pain as the primary concern. However, if the research is really so benign, why substitute other sentient animals for humans in "pain-free" experiments? Why not use humans? One reason is that some of the subjects are killed, albeit in a merciful fashion, after the experiment. (Eventually, all are slated to be killed when they are no longer useful for research). A second is that there may be long-term damages from the interventions. Another is that even the most benign intervention robs the subjects of living in their natural surroundings and doing what they would want to do in such surroundings. With many experiments humans would have to leave the comforts of their home and regular life and live, at least for a period, in laboratory-like conditions.

What we are apparently left with is the basic claim that medical research on other animals is justified because humans are superior to, and therefore more precious than other animals. It is only appropriate for humans, then, to demand the sacrifice of lesser creatures for their benefit -- similar to how gods were once considered entitled to human sacrifice. The ways that humans are superior are many, but the same case could be made for any other species—each is distinctly better in some ways in doing certain things or in adapting to various situations. As Bernard Rollin[2] says, if one were to select such things as differential reproduction, species longevity, and adaptability "both humans and rats lose hands-down to the cockroach."

Notwithstanding, because of our written and spoken language, we have been able to pass on and accumulate knowledge of all kinds and complexities, and to improve the speed of communication to the point where it is virtually instant. We are superior to all other forms of life in a tremendous variety of ways. However, this "superiority" is suspect. We have also been inventive as to how to destroy life – be it by radiation, toxic chemicals, or the gradual pollution of our environment so that it will, perhaps not so far in the future, be unsustainable for all.

There are serious problems with our social systems also. We have allowed ourselves to increase our numbers so that in many places in the world it is impossible for many, perhaps most, of the inhabitants to sustain their existence without periodic, increasingly frequent, donations of basic sustenance. And we may seem to be unable to control this increase of population and the subsequent depletion of resources. Even in well-off countries, where, at least for the present generation, there is enough for all, the distribution of wealth is so unequal that many live in dire poverty. The gap between the "haves" and the "have nots" is getting larger. Hardly a description of a "superior" social system. Considering how we use our knowledge of things and how we distribute our resources, it is clear that we have become a danger to not only ourselves but to all life on our planet.

All of the theories that justify experimenting on other animals for our benefit do so on the basis of humans somehow being of greater worth than other animals, which worth is generally thought of in terms of being superior to them.   Once we question the "goodness" of that "superiority we undermine the whole justification structure.

The fact of the matter is that the human species, as a collective, has accumulated the knowledge and the means to dominate most other animal species (except "pests" such as cockroaches and human head lice).   It is this superiority, that of power, which ultimately supports medical research that uses animals as human surrogates. And as Rollin[2] points out: "If superior means that we are more powerful than other creatures and can in fact do as we wish to them, this is surely true but has no moral relevance.   To say that it has is to affirm that might makes right and to destroy morality altogether."

But, you could ask, does not might carry with it a certain moral authority, especially when that might has been gained by legitimate means?   Humans have developed tremendous power in that they have developed a system of passing on power to each other through what one could call "tools."   However, those who possess the tools, whether a computer or a simple hammer, or money inherited from others, don't have to know anything about how to actually make the tool, only how to use it.   This would seem to undercut the argument that everyone who can use a tool has some special moral authority to use it as they will.   This is certainly not true with weapons.

Still, does not the system itself confer moral authority on those who are part of it?   Perhaps the best way to respond to this claim is to consider another, totally different sort of might, one that is well known to those in the realm of medicine - the ability of cancer, viruses, and bacteria to "recreate" themselves in response to threatening changes in their environment, whether human-made or natural.   This protean response has, by and large, met and matched all the technological advances of modern medicine.   If it is obvious that this form of might is amoral, it should also be obvious to us that might, in and of itself, is amoral.   Morality and ethics are created by the introduction of the concepts of concern and responsibility for the effects of our actions on other entities.   The only way to be truly "superior" to other forms of life is to act in an ethical manner towards them and among ourselves.   This, like all other capacities, wastes away if not practiced.

It has been asked, however, whether there isn't some evolutionary point in the complexity of life where it doesn't make sense to talk about treating a form of life in a moral or ethical manner.   If so, then might and right are on different axes.   Surely, we do not have to worry about treating amoebas in a moral way, or plants, or creatures, such as ants, whose lives appear to be completely preprogrammed?   Yes and no.   It all depends on the context.   If something is of value, then even "things" should be treated with care.   For example, a mountain may be an essential part of a habitat that sustains many forms of life, and to allow mining of it for minerals would harm the habitat. In this way, at least, even things such as mountains have legal rights, as law professor Christopher Stone[14] so aptly argues. It can be illegal and is unethical to change a mountain in such a way as to harm the habitat it supports without some overriding greater good. From an environmental point of view, it is hard to find a "greater good."

This consideration is not irrelevant to our concern in this chapter: the moral status of animals. Within the environmental point of view this book takes, animals, even ants, are certainly entitled to special protection from experimentation which could threaten the continuation of the species. Species diversity is vital to a sustainable environment. The situation is better now, but at one time, primate research was being conducted even at the risk of depleting the numbers of threatened or endangered species.

The ability to feel, and, beyond that, sufficient consciousness of one's existence to be able to have and pursue interests, are also generally considered important characteristics of creatures to be protected. This value can be imputed by us, or, as argued by Holmes Rolston[15] in his book on environmental ethics, as somehow inherent in other creatures, or, as both. Regardless, we accept these demarcation points of ability to feel and to pursue individual interests, albeit that they are imprecise, given our inability to "get beneath the skin" of other creatures and discover what they feel and think. We cannot even do that with other members of our own species. .

There is one more argument defending current practices, perhaps the crucial one. As a way of gently introducing it, let us enjoy an actual account that shows all too well the jumble of attitudes we have towards other animals. This will be followed by an another important background factor, the monetary commitment medical science has made towards this method of research,

MICE AND MEN IN AN ANIMAL RESEARCH LAB

Harold Herzog[16] of Western Carolina University has taken to take a humorous view of the way we consider and treat other animals. He notes that human attitudes towards other species "are often based on emotional criteria such as how cute they are and how we define their social roles."

In an earlier article, Herzog[17] provides an amusing and instructive example of the inconsistencies in our attitudes. The setting is the Walters Life Sciences Building at the University of Tennessee, a typical university animal research laboratory. This multimillion dollar facility hosts about 15,000 mice in any given year. The vast preponderance of the mice are "good" mice, good in that they "sacrifice their lives for what researchers hope will be the betterment of the human condition." Accordingly, they are afforded the care and protection mandated by the US Department of Agriculture.

And then there are the "bad" mice. These are the mice who escaped their confined spaces and now roam freely around the building. They are bad not only in that they set a poor example, but because they infect the good mice with whatever diseases they pick up, and this interferes with the planned experiments. Attempts to eliminate these mice with poisons were discarded for fear that the good mice might also be contaminated, and snap traps were found to be ineffective. Sticky traps, left in the preferred routes of the bad mice, became the method of choice. The mice frequently are found dead by the time the traps are collected and those who aren't are gassed while still stuck to the trap. Herzog doubts that an experiment in which mice were glued to pieces of cardboard until they died would receive approval from most animal care committees. Thus, although the mice are of the same species as the good mice, they are given a lower moral status, one not deserving of any protection.

Still another category of mice, with still another moral status, is "feeder mice." Among the other experimental animals in the research lab are snakes, lizards, and large toads. They are fed mice as part of their diets. Yet such predators are otherwise generally considered of lower moral status than warm-blooded mice.

It is not inconceivable that one of the mice would become a pet. In fact, Herzog's son had a mouse for a pet for two years, which, as such, received solicitous, affectionate care until it died. It was then ceremonially buried in a flower garden, complete with a tombstone.

However, there are also "bad" mice in households, even in Herzog's, and snap traps are set to catch them.

This story illustrates the fact that the attitude of the vast majority of humans towards other animals is not founded on some rational, justifiable theory but rather on whether an animal is attractive or repulsive to them or whether it furthers or frustrates their goals. The implementation of this attitude in medical research, in product testing, and in school science labs is a growing, multibillion dollar business. Back in 1982 about six billion dollars was spent for medical research in the USA, much of it for animal research.[18] By 1996 this had grown to 17 billion dollars (excluding research and development).[19] By comparison, the total federal outlay in 1998 for pollution control and abatement was $6.6 billion.[20] Millions of animals are involved in medical research, and they require hundreds of facilities to breed and house them while awaiting experimentation. Scores of thousands of jobs are also involved, many of which are prestigious and well paid. In Switzerland, alone, the pharmaceutical industry reacted to a national initiative to eliminate experimentation on other animals by claiming it would lead to the elimination of 10,000 jobs.[21]

This provides the context for the final argument, the one that seems to be the basic sustaining motivation for the animals-for-humans research industry, once we strip away all the scientific and moral wrappings.

Humans have a right to defend themselves and to promote other self-interests they consider vital, cost what it may, in terms of other animals. The right to self-defense is well known as a civil right. It provides a defense against murder of another human being and certainly of other animals, even the last one of a species, providing that it was, apparently, the only way of defending one's own life. A related right is that of self-interest. The pedigree of supporters of these arguments includes the philosophical giant, Emmanuel Kant. In his exposition of the Categorical Imperative, Kant[22] noted that individuals have an "indirect" duty to secure their own happiness. "For discomfort with one's condition . . . might easily become *a great temptation to transgression of duty.*" In his *Metaphysic of Ethics*, Kant[23] pointed out that owing a duty to one's self is not a contradiction, rather just an extension of the imposition on ourselves of all ethical duties. Among the self-duties he mentions, one is primary, namely the commandment, "Know Thyself," which is described as being sensitive to one's conscience. More recently, philosopher John Thomas[24] notes: "In fact we do have moral duties to ourselves. . ." The one he specifically mentions is self-protection.

Now, there are no end of things which could be claimed under the egress of "securing one's happiness," and obviously this "indirect duty" must be bounded in some way. Kant binds it by restricting its use to insuring that one does not default on one's other duties, and by making the supreme self-duty that of being true to one's conscience. Self-protection seems to be the most secure way of interpreting this duty but it, too, needs bounding. Let us see how far this notion that of self-protection or self-defense will take us in defending medical research using other animals for humans.

We will start with perhaps the simplest expression of this "right" to self-defense: the right to fight for one's job, or conversely, the right to defend oneself from being laid off. Certainly, to the extent that such a right exists, it should apply to workers in animal laboratories as well as to any other job holders. Yet, this must be put in a greater context in order to judge its legitimacy. Does the person who has the job really need it to have enough for basic existence and to maintain their psychological equilibrium and that of their family? Can the person probably find other employment that would meet such basic needs? And finally, do the duties performed in the job harm others? If the latter is the case, the job is transgressing on the rights of others and the case must be made that the right to this particular type of job is justified in terms of the harm caused. Normally, we concern ourselves with harm to other humans, but we do not have to limit ourselves to this realm. Here, the harm is direct to animals who are substituted for humans in experiments. There is also indirect harm done to humans and other living beings insofar as the research leads to misleading results and to overly expensive treatments which siphon off resources from other, more important, societal and planetary needs.

In some cases the threatened loss is not that of basic employment but rather that of fame and fortune. Here, the case for self-protection is weaker, being more a loss of "privileges" rather than of the means for basic sustenance. That does not mean that scientists who experience such a threat will not fight hard, and with great skill, to maintain their position. How well people are able to defend job positions is usually not a matter of how truly threatened they are but how elevated their positions are and what skills they possess for convincing others.

Another group of people who may feel the need for self-protection are those who are ill with a currently incurable disease or suffer under some crippling handicap. They may fight for the hope of a cure, and, if they believe this hope will be diminished by virtue of reduction of any kind of medical research, they, and those concerned about them, will lobby hard for its continuation, indeed, for even more resources to be given for such research. Understandable as this stance is, hope of a cure or for substantial amelioration of one's condition is prime for manipulation by others. They can use such hope as a way of getting funding for research which really has only a small chance of being successful. As such, it is a rather insubstantial basis in comparison to that of harm to other causes that lack funding and support.

So we now come to the crucial question of these last two chapters: if we apply the environmental-social justice point of view rather than the prevailing parochial one, would medical research that substitutes animals for humans be considered a vital, necessary aspect of medical research?

Due to the leap of faith required to cross the species gap, the case for research on animals for the benefit of humans is inherently weak; thus medical research of this kind must have an especially high value to be privileged in <u>any</u> distribution of resources, even from a parochial point of view. One does not need such preliminary, investigative research to greatly improve the offerings of the medical industry; one needs only the kind of research that determines which are the best ways to implement and distribute fairly those services that are already available and of known value.

It should also be noted that from an environmental, planetary perspective we have done wrong. By considering ourselves as more worthy than other species, we have not only become more of a bane than

a blessing to almost all other forms of life, but we threaten our own future. Substituting other animals for humans in medical research reinforces this destructive attitude. This provides one more reason for severely restricting this practice.

The chances for doing so may well be slim, given the powerful financial and professional incentives for continuing this methodology. However, the emergence of cheaper, more effective alternatives, alternatives that do not sacrifice other animals, erodes substantially the financial motive, and could lead to a reappraisal of the basic methodology, itself.

Proposed standards on substitution of other animals for humans in research intended to benefit humans

XIV	Animals whose species would be threatened by experimentation on them should not be substituted for humans in research intended to benefit humans.
	Maintaining the diversity of species is vital to providing a livable environment for all current and future humans and other forms of life.

XV	Sentient life forms who are capable of having and pursuing individual interests should not be substituted for humans in research intended to benefit humans.
	Neither the scientific nor the ethical basis for this sort of experimentation justifies its continued use. Due to over two million years of evolutionary differentiation, other animals make inadequate substitutes for humans in determining the results of any intervention on humans, as demonstrated by the unanticipated, sometimes devastating, adverse side effects of many drugs. Also, development of alternative techniques have progressed to the point where they can, by and large, be substituted for humans in preliminary investigations.
	The ethical justification lacks substance and consistency. In the final analysis, it resolves into a "we have the might, therefore we have the right" position, and a form of self-defense for those in, or connected to, the animal research industry.
	If the case is strong enough for trying out a particular intervention, humans can be found who would submit to the intervention, and the results from these experiments would much better determine the reliable effects of the experimental substance or procedure on humans than is now the case.
	All subjects should be fully informed and fully voluntary. Exceptions might only be made with respect to humans whose state is such that they are unable to give their consent and the hazards of the conventional intervention are as great or greater than those of the experimental intervention.

This is the last of the Proposed standards.

Below is a summary of the others.

| I | In conducting cost analyses of medical interventions, short-term reductions in cost of care that may result from the intervention shall not be counted as "savings" and subtracted from the costs of the intervention, since they are only postponed costs, not real savings. Exceptions could be made for chronic conditions and diseases since they could involve real savings. |

| II | In determining whether or not public funding should be involved in the research (or treatment) phase of an intervention, the following criterion is proposed: The expense for each extended Quality-Adjusted Life Year (QALY) should be calculated. It should be less than the average yearly expenditures that are required to adequately maintain a minimally-sized family in a well-off country; namely, a family that contains one parent and one child under 18. Research which can be anticipated with reasonable certainty to result in products and procedures which would exceed this amount should not be supported with public funding. The amount includes the cost of the initial intervention and any continuing treatment associated with it throughout the life of the individual. As an example, in the USA the average amount expended by a single-parent, single-child family unit in 1995 was estimated to be $22,626 (US Bureau of the Census, 1998, Table 735, p. 466). This would be approximately $25,000 in 2000. Thus, in the USA no public funding would support research that could be anticipated to result in an intervention that would exceed $25,000 per QALY. The same restriction would apply to already existing interventions. Whether $22,626 was adequate in 1995 to insure a reasonable chance of living a satisfying life and making a positive contribution to the society for each member of the family is not known. If inadequate, and one would suspect as much since it is only $3,236 more than the average amount expended by single persons, this is hardly a reason to increase the ethical allotment to the most well-endowed sector of the economy (Table 734, p. 465). |

III   No "straw men" comparisons Trial studies should be designed in such a way as to compare the experimental procedures and products to one or more robust alternative treatments, if such exist, and not to weak versions of them. When the alternative treatment is "standard medical practice," it should not be some weak version of it, but rather one which the physicians and other personnel are carefully instructed in what is recommended practice.

If this standard is not observed it is impossible to determine how much, if any, the intervention adds to what can already be accomplished by following recommended practice.

IV   In any nonpreliminary study, use both single-cause and all-cause mortality as main end points in any intervention that purports to be life extending. Do not settle for surrogate end points, even if combined with a mortality end point, since this negates the value of the end point.

Surrogate end points have been found to be inadequate and to lead to adoption of intervention with unknown, even deadly effects. Hence they are to be avoided as main end points in any final assessments of life-extending interventions. Combining them with mortality in a main end point only obscures the results as to actual effects on mortality and lends itself to abuse by those who wish to promote a particular intervention when the surrogate end point(s) are more promising than the mortality end points.

V   Use all-reported treatment in determining any change in quality of life due to interventions that are intended to be primarily ameliorative in nature.

To truly determine the degree, extent, and nature of side effects of any intervention, it is insufficient to merely look at the effects that are obviously connected to it, such as the effects on the morbidity of that particular disease, since other disease processes may be triggered by the intervention. Also trauma could result, such as a fall or an automobile accident caused by dizziness which is a side effect of the drug. Hence, it is necessary to determine, as much as possible, all the postintervention treatments that patients report or their records reveal, i.e., all-reported treatment.

| **VI** | Use all-cause mortality and all-reported treatment in the calculation of Quality-Adjusted Life Years gained.
                             Only a full accounting of all intervention effects can result in an accurate measuring of QALYs. |

| **VII** | No early termination of studies for less than truly good reasons. Ongoing studies should not be cut short before the full term solely for the reason that a statistically significant result has been reached for a main end point. They should be stopped only if the proportional difference is obviously of clinical significance (for example, the incidence of permanent disability or the number of deaths are clearly higher in one group and there seems to be no other plausible explanation for that).
Stopping a trial early is a judgment call that lends itself to bias in favor of what the investigators had hoped to prove was true. It stops short any correction to the results that would occur if there were a reversal of the findings in the later stage of the study. |

| **VIII** | All clinical trials should be registered in an easily accessible, public, international registry.
Reviewers and those who wish to conduct meta-analyses or other aggregate analyses on studies need to identify those trials that led to multiple publications. Information about trials that were not published or completed would also provide useful information for other overview purposes. |

IX   Disclosure. Both the funding source(s) for any paper and any financial ties to commercial firms of all investigators in any study should be disclosed to potential publishers and, if the paper is published, this information should also be divulged to readers in a prominent place.

Without such information editors and reviewers, and later the intended readers, are not in a position to judge for themselves the likelihood of commercial bias in the design or write-up of the paper. There are many other kinds of biases, such as favoritism of certain academic institutions, theories, and types of research, but this one is more powerful than others due to its pervasiveness in First World societies where most medical research is done.

X   All major players in the publishing process -- reviewers, editors, and any others who have a say in the final judgment in the acceptance of a paper or book for publication should:

A. Disclose any financial conflict of interest that might affect their judgment on the decision. This would include any occasional or continuing consultancy or other employment, paid presentations, expense covered trips to   conferences, and stock holdings of themselves or family   members. In addition:

B. Reviewers should be selected who do not have any such conflict of interest.

C. Editors, being the primary gatekeepers of the publishing world, should divest themselves of conflicting financial interests, and failing that, withdraw from the decision-making process on any submitted paper in which they have a financial interest.

XI In the abstract or any other prominent place where statistical results are reported, the results between the intervention and the nonintervention group(s) should be expressed primarily in absolute terms, not in terms of relative reductions in risks. Alternative absolute risk-derived measures, such as Number Needed to Treat (NNT), would also be appropriate for prominent placement.

Relative-risk reduction, while perhaps necessary or useful for statistical manipulations or comparisons, is a misleading statistic for most readers and for the mass media. It provides an exaggerated impression of the efficacy of an intervention.

XII No industry-affiliated ghost writers. Assistance from ghost writers for research articles, editorials, and commentaries — either in professional journals or intended for the mass media — should be acknowledged and/or otherwise compensated. Offers from commercial interests to supply writing assistance should be rejected.

XIII Unbiased publication of all worthy studies and commentaries. Medical journals and other professional publications should institute procedures to insure that articles which are promotive of new products or procedures do not receive more favorable treatment — such as better chance of publication or quicker publication — than those that are critical of products or procedures.

This would mean, for example, that papers that claim statistically significant results would not be more likely to be published or published any sooner than papers that find that the intervention does not show any statistically significant advantage over the comparison treatment, or lack of treatment.

Also, the editors should critically review all articles submitted for publication to insure that the titles, abstracts, presentation of results, and citation of relevant literature do not distort the likely impact of the article in favor of a commercial or institutional interest.

References

[1] Malone TE (1992). The moral imperative for biological research. In: Porter RJ, Malone TE, eds. *Biomedical research: collaboration and conflict of interest.* Baltimore: The Johns Hopkins University Press: 3-32.

[2] Rollin BE (August, 1985). The moral status of research animals in psychology. *American Psychologist*: 920-26.

[3] Loeb JM, Hendee WR, et al. (1989). In defense of animal research. *JAMA* 262: 2716-20.

[4] Leopold A (1987). *A Sand County Almanac.* New York: Oxford University Press: 224.

[5] Loew FM. (1989). Animals in research. In: Beauchamp TL, Walters L, eds. *Contemporary issues in bioethics.* Belmont, CA: Wadsworth Publishing Company: 301-12.

[6] McClosky HJ (1989). The moral case for experimentation on animals. In: Beauchamp TL, Walters L, eds. *Contemporary issues in bioethics.* Belmont, CA: Wadsworth Publishing Company: 485-65.

[7] Brody BA (1998). *The ethics of biomedical research: An international perspective.* New York: Oxford University Press.

[8] ibid. p.16.

[9] Perkins KA (November, 1990). Support of animal research needed: Comment on Dewsbury. *American Psychologist*: 1270-71.

[10] Novak MA (July, 1991). Psychologists care deeply about animals. *American Psychological Association Monitor*: 4.

[11] Vanderberg HL (ed) (1996). *The ethics of research involving human subjects: Facing the 21st century* (Appendices A, B, and C). Frederick, MD: University Publishing Group.

[12] Kaufman S (May 24, 2000). Personal communication made in pursuit of reviewing the chapter.

[13] Koshland DE. (1989). Animal rights and animal wrongs. *Science*: 243: 1253.

[14] Stone CD (1987). *Earth and other ethics. The case for moral pluralism.* New York: Harper Row.

[15] Rolston H (1988). *Environmental ethics.* Philadelphia: Temple University Press.

[16] Herzog HA. (March, 1991). Conflicts of interests: Kittens and boa constrictors, pets and research. *American Psychologist*: 246-47.

[17] Herzog HA (June,1988). The moral status of mice. *American Psychologist*: 473-74.

[18] Colen BD (1986). *Hard choices: mixed blessings of modern medical technology.* New York: G. P. Putman's Sons.

[19] US Bureau of the Census (1998). *Statistical abstract of the United States* (118th edition, Table 165). Washington, DC.

[20] CQ Staff (1998, February 8). How each agency and department would fare under Clinton budget. *Congressional Quarterly*: 297-313.

[21] Tiershutz-Initiative bedroht 10,000 Stellen (February 19,1992). *Swiss-American Review*: 2.

[22] Kant I(1929). *Kant Selections*. 1929. New York: Charles Schribner's Sons.

[23] KantI (1886). *The metaphysic of ethics.* Edinburgh: T.T. Clark

[24] Thomas J (November 23,1987). The professional and the moral life. An address at the annual meeting of the Western Association of Counselor Educators and Supervisors in Portland, OR, USA.

Chapter Seven

How To Make A Mountain And A Mint Out Of, At Most, A Molehill: Statin Drugs

Andrew Thompson, Norman J. Temple

Blessed is he who expects nothing, for he shall never be disappointed.
Alexander Pope, 1725[1]

Practices of unknown value account for a sizable portion of the increased expense of modern medicine. Some of them involve the use of expensive diagnostic procedures and equipment, which, once in place, require being used to justify their cost. Other procedures seem innocuously inexpensive but are so often and widely administered that the total cost of using them is considerable.

This chapter begins our review of some medical interventions which already cost huge sums of money, are expanding in use, and are of dubious value. These don't begin to tap the repertoire of such practices; rather, they represent the tip of the iceberg. Whole books could and should be written detailing other such abuses of resources. But the examples here should provide an indication of their nature and breadth. At the end of each chapter we will evaluate the research that has been done by comparison with the Proposed Standards.

We will start with a fad-like test, examine its justification, and then look at the research supporting the drug treatment that is often prescribed when one gets a "bad score" on the test.

Most of us are familiar with the following "facts": total cholesterol over the low 200s mg/dL is bad, over 300 is worse, and over 400 is terrible (or 5.2, 7.8, and 10.4 mmol/l, respectively). Also, it is bad if the LDL (low-density lipoprotein) component is more than six times higher than the HDL (high-density lipoprotein) level since that accelerates atherosclerosis. Eat less foods containing saturated fat and cholesterol to lower your cholesterol levels. Raise HDL, the "good" lipoprotein, by exercise. If diet doesn't work, take drugs.

A. Thompson and N.J. Temple (eds.), Ethics, Medical Research, and Medicine, 95–116.
© 2001 *Kluwer Academic Publishers. Printed in the Netherlands.*

A complex set of assertions simply stated and repeated so often that it has become a truism. What hasn't been emphasized is that things are far from being that simple. Each assertion is a generalization that doesn't always hold true and the scientists don't know why.

An immediate result of the cholesterol hypothesis, namely, that too much cholesterol, especially of the "bad kind," leads to heart disease, is that measurement of cholesterol in the blood is an "in" thing. No age, from childhood on, is spared from such investigation. Some of this testing is done primarily for research purposes but there seems to be an underlying assumption that if it is a valuable test for any group or age it must be for all. A task force established by the US National Heart, Lung, and Blood Institute, for example, has recommended that all adults, 21 and over, know their cholesterol levels. Perhaps, as a result of this recommendation, some college campuses periodically offer free testing to all students. Inexpensive as such testing is per person, if this policy were to be extended to all young adults in the USA, the cost would reach into the billions of dollars, given that there are about 80 million men aged 20 to 35 and women aged 20 to 45.[2]

This recommendation for early testing was discredited by a group of outside experts who concurred that cholesterol testing and treatment is of potential value only beginning in middle age (35 and over for men and 45 and over for women). They claimed that starting a diet and drug therapy at those points will provide all the benefits to be obtained from such treatment.[2]

It could be argued that such testing would be of value to young adults with high levels of cholesterol if it persuaded them to start healthy diets. But the hazard of this approach is that all those who do not have a high cholesterol level may use the results as confirmation that they are immune from the effects of their bad eating habits and otherwise unhealthy lifestyles. This is simply not true. For one thing, most people who develop coronary heart disease (CHD) do not have a high total cholesterol level.[3] Also, healthy lifestyles have a preventive value for many diseases, not just heart disease.

Routine testing at older ages also doesn't make much sense, according to a British study. It involved 21,520 men aged 35-64 and compared the death rate from CHD of men who had been selected to have their cholesterol tested to that of matched controls five to ten years after the experimental group had been screened. Their conclusion stated[4]:

> *. . . screening for IHD [CHD] is not effective. If the false positive rate [rate of number of participants falsely thought to be at risk of IHD based on the screening] were set at 5 percent, total cholesterol alone would identify 12 percent of future IHD deaths, apo B [a protein also measured by cholesterol testing] alone would identify 17 percent, and the most efficient*

combination of total cholesterol, apolipoproteins, blood pressure, smoking, and family history would identify no more than 30 percent. . . If the remedy were to recommend lifestyle changes (diet, smoking cessation, and exercise) that apply to the whole population, then screening would serve no purpose. It might even do harm, as the vast majority of the population . . . would be judged screen-negative and could take false reassurance and be less inclined to adopt the lifestyle changes, yet three-quarters of IHD deaths would occur in screen-negative people.

Treatment, whenever it begins, is frequently based on the hypothesis that total cholesterol levels ought to be lowered to around 200 mg/dL. However, the relationship between cholesterol levels and arterial clogging is very complex and far from completely understood. Any given component of what is commonly measured when determining cholesterol levels -- HDL, LDL, and triglycerides -- serves a different theoretical role and each, and the formula-derived total amount, is used as an indicator of arterial health. But none of the components or the total is a sure indicator. In fact, there are many different factors that are thought to influence the deterioration of heart arteries.[5]

Diet and exercise strategies have been very successful in lowering both mortality from CHD and overall mortality. Diets commonly used for this purpose have been very restrictive of fat intake, especially saturated fat, and include at least 400 grams (about 14 ounces) of fruits and vegetables, or are supplemented with fish oils.[6,7, 8,9,10] In most people, depending on the dietary change, they also lower cholesterol levels. But this only explains part of the success for these diets. Other factors most probably involved are antioxidant vitamins, high-fiber content, omega-3 fats, and potassium.

However, there is no profit to the pharmaceutical industry if dietary changes are implemented. This may be why so much research has been expended in the development and trial of cholesterol-lowering drugs and so little in designing programs that would encourage and implement the establishment of healthy diet and exercise patterns, both as prevention and as treatment. What we have instead is a wide choice of drugs that lower various components of cholesterol as well as the total amount for most people. These levels are surrogate end points: lowering them does not necessarily improve the overall health of the individual. The only way to determine actual benefit is to use the Proposed Standard end points of all-cause mortality and reportable-cause morbidity, as explained in chapter three.

Let us now review the studies that have been used to support the use of cholesterol-lowering drugs. Do they truly do so or are they examples of the saying: "If you torture the data long enough, it will eventually confess?" It is not an idle question. Largely because of these studies, or rather because of how they were interpreted and presented to the professional and general public, the prescription of such drugs increased from £20 million in 1993 to over £113 million in 1997 in Great Britain.[11] In the USA annual sales increased 29 percent in 1997 to $3.7 billion or more than half as much as the total federal outlay, $6.7 billion, for training and employment in that year.[12,13]

1.REVIEW OF STUDIES

We can divide the cholesterol-lowering drugs into two groups: the pre-4S (Scandinavian Simvastatin Survival Study)[14,15] and the post-4S studies. Ravnskov's work, mentioned in chapter three in our discussion of citation bias, is relevant here also. He reviewed 22 of the pre-4S "controlled" cholesterol-lowering studies. These studies are the best science has to offer at this point in that they randomly assign patients to experimental and placebo groups. He found publication bias, citation bias, and suspect statistics - all of which worked to the advantage of those promoting the drugs.

He also found that the experimenters claimed that the studies were set up so that no one treating the patients or collecting the data would know which patients were taking the drug and which the placebo. This is called "blinding" of the medical staff and data analysts and is important to do since "unblinded" studies, studies in which those who administer the treatment or those who analyze the results, know which patients are in which group, have been found to be biased. Apparently, administrators and analysts unconsciously or consciously act in such a way as to promote treatment-favorable results.[16] Of particular importance in this regard is the fact that some of these cholesterol-lowering drugs have obvious side effects, thus making it quite apparent to the medical personnel which patients were taking them.[17]

Only two studies lasted longer than five years (one of 11 years and one of 9.6 years) and they provided one partial drug-supportive result and two negative ones. Only the supportive finding was cited frequently. The "support" of most of the allegedly supportive shorter studies dissipated when analyzed by conventional statistics. Ravnskov[17] concluded that: "lowering serum cholesterol concentrations does not reduce mortality and is unlikely to prevent coronary heart disease. Claims of the opposite are based on preferential citation of supportive trials."

The drug industry was well aware of such findings and aware of the fact that some experts were concerned. So, simultaneously with continuing to promote the array of cholesterol-reducing drugs that they offered at the time, they continued the search for ones that could make a better case for being both safe and effective. The 4S study on patients with known coronary disease gave them what they wanted: a statistically significant difference in favor of the group that took the drug, not only in reduced mortality from CHD but also in mortality from all causes.[15] Let us now take a look at this study and the five others that have built the foundation on which the cholesterol-lowering industry now stands. None of the studies replicated the others: each focused on a different population, albeit overlapping to some degree. Lacking such replication of findings, especially from an industry-independent source, no definitive conclusion should be reached about any of the findings on any of the populations. Each of the studies involved several thousand subjects. This is required if statistically significant differences are to be expected with rather modest actual differences.

The Scandinavian Simvastatin Survival Study Group (the "4S Study")

The 4S study enrolled 4,444 patients (3,617 males and 827 females), with a mean age of about 59 years. All patients had known coronary disease and a total cholesterol level of 212 to 309 mg/dl (5.5 to 8.0 mmol/l). Hence, they were at a high risk for death due to CHD and of death in general. The selection of high-risk patients was necessary since one of the goals of the study was to determine if the statin drug would be effective in lowering the rate of all-cause morality within the time period of three years or until such time as total mortality reached 440 deaths.[14,15]

The West of Scotland Coronary Prevention Study Group (the "WOSCPS Study")

The WOSCPS study enrolled 6,595 men aged 45 to 64, with a mean age of 55. They had no known CHD but did have high total cholesterol levels of 259 to 295 mg/dl (6.4 to 7.6 mmol/l). Hence, they were a group who were at high risk of developing CHD and the purpose of the study was to determine if the statin drug would reduce the incidence of the combined end points of nonfatal heart attacks and death from CHD. This was determined at the end of five years of treatment.[18,19]

The Cholesterol and Recurrent Events Study: Parts 1 and 2 (CARE 1 and 2)

The CARE study enrolled patients aged 50 to 75 who had heart disease and only average levels of total cholesterol (below 240 or 6.2 mmol/l) and low-density lipoprotein (LDL) levels of 115 to 174 (3.0 to 4.5 mmol/l). For purposes of analysis the participants were divided into a younger group of 4,159 subjects (3,583 men and 576 women) aged 50 to 68 (CARE 1), and an older group of 1,283 subjects (238 women and 1,045 men) aged 65 to 75 (CARE 2). Why the overlap in age is not clear. Both studies were intended to determine if the statin drug used would reduce damage from heart disease in patients with average cholesterol levels. Both studies followed the patients for five years. CARE 1 did so by choosing the combined incidence of fatal coronary events and nonfatal heart attacks as its main end point (main outcome criterion).[3] CARE 2 choose a broad band of primary end points: coronary death, nonfatal heart attacks, angioplasty or bypass surgery, and stroke.[20]

The Air Force/Texas Coronary Atherosclerosis Prevention Study (AFCAPS/TexCAPS)

This study enrolled 6,605 civilians and active or retired military personnel from an air force base and a medical center in Texas. There were 5,608 men, with an average age of 58, and 997 women, with an average age of 62. The participants had no known heart disease and had normal to mildly elevated total cholesterol levels and reduced high-density lipoprotein levels. The study was intended to determine if the statin drug used would significantly lower the incidence of sudden cardiac death, fatal and nonfatal heart attacks, and unstable angina, even of generally healthy individuals with near normal cholesterol levels.[21,22]

The Long-term Intervention with Pravastatin in Ischaemic Disease study (the LIPID Study)

The LIPID study enrolled 9014 patients with a history of acute heart attacks or unstable angina and with moderate to high total cholesterol levels. There were 1,511 women and 7,503 men aged 31 to 75 with an average age of 62. The primary end point was death from CHD, measured over a time period averaging 6.1 years.[23,24] The physicians were not blinded to who were receiving the statin drug or the placebo but "were uncertain of the long-terms benefits of cholesterol lowering."[23]

APPLICATION OF THE PROPOSED STANDARDS TO THE RESEARCH DESIGN OF THE STUDIES

Proposed Standards I and II: Costs

It would have been remarkable if any of the studies had fully incorporated cost-effectiveness in their design, one that recorded costs of treatment other than from CHD. When most of the studies were initiated, the awareness of the need for cost-benefit analysis was not high and the pressure to do them was low. And from a commercial point of view, why find out something which might be used against prescribing your product? However, by the time the studies were completed there was more awareness and more pressure so some post hoc, cost-effectiveness analyses were done. We will report on them a little later when we apply the Proposed Standards for cost to these studies. The LIPID study is perhaps an exception: it does list a cost-effectiveness committee but reported no data from its efforts. Presumably, this will come later.

Proposed Standard III: Disclosure of Conflicts of Interest

All of the studies were supported by the drug companies that produced the drugs being studied. Information about other ties to these companies by the investigators or the data analysts is typically lacking, and, even when offered, is almost always in small print and is often difficult to locate. This is what we could find:

The 4S study notes, in a long list of the contributors who performed the study, that an employee of the drug company was responsible for the analysis of the data.

The WOSCPS study lists some individuals who served as "liaisons" to the sponsor. It does not acknowledge other potential conflicts of interest, although the later cost-effectiveness study by Caro et al[25] indicates that the first author and chair of the executive committee, John Shepherd, as "advising" the drug company "from time to time."

The two CARE studies do not provide information of this sort.

A paper on the AFCAPS/TexCAPS study lists authors who were employed by the drug company as regular employees, as consultants, as speakers, and as researchers in other studies by the firm. Five of ten the authors were so employed.[22]

The LIPID study declares that the members of the Safety and Data Monitoring Committee had no affiliation with the sponsor. It makes no such statement about the investigators.

Proposed Standard IV: "Straw men" or "robust alternative" treatment?

All of the studies chose as their comparison treatment the administration of a placebo, under what is described as "standard practice" conditions for both groups. The question arises as to whether this standard practice was designed to hide or to reveal the distinct role of the experimental medication? If you wish to maximize the chances that the drug will be found to have positive effects, even though it adds nothing, or may even add a negative element, to what already exists in recommended interventions, then you choose a weak, straw man version of standard practice. If, however, you want to find out if the drug will add anything, or much, of value to what could be achieved without it, then you choose a strong, robust version of standard practice, one that incorporates all the wisdom at the moment as how best to treat such patients. After all, why prescribe a new drug if what could be done for the patient could be done just as well, if not better, by simply following recommended practice?

All of the statin studies failed the "robust standard practice" test in two respects — how they implemented dietary measures and their prescription of other, known and recommended medications.

Dietary Measures

All of the studies had available to them medical standards published in 1987 in Europe and 1988 in the USA. Both sets of standards recommend dietary counseling, preferably by dietitians, before any drug therapy for heart disease is started. The European standards recommend dietary management as "necessary for all primary hyperlipidemias" (high levels of fats in the blood) and as the "sole therapy for the majority of persons with elevated levels. . .A dietitian, supported by the patient's physician, is best able to instruct the patient, adapt the diet to energy needs and food preferences, and (if response is inadequate) to monitor ongoing compliance."[26] The US National Cholesterol Education Program (NCEP) states unequivocally[27]:

> *Drug therapy is likely to continue for many years, or for a lifetime. Hence, the decision to add drug therapy to the regimen should be made only after vigorous efforts at dietary treatment have not proven sufficient.*

"Vigorous efforts" are defined as "a minimum of six months of intensive dietary counseling" prior to initiating drug therapy. This is to occur in two steps. First, a Step One Diet is introduced. This reduces the intake of total fat to less than 30 percent of calories, saturated fat to less than ten percent of calories, and cholesterol to less than 300 mg per day. If that doesn't bring down the cholesterol levels sufficiently, then a Step Two Diet is initiated which lowers the saturated fat to less than seven percent of the total calories and the cholesterol to less than 200 mg per day. "Involvement of a registered dietitian is very useful, particularly for intensive dietary therapy such as the Step Two Diet." Let us see how closely the statin studies followed these recommendations.

The 4S study reports that it followed the 1987 recommendations of the European Atherosclerosis Society. However, the study design provides no specifics as to who provided the dietary advice (intended to lower total fat intake to less than 30 percent), how often, and how vigorously, only that patients were given eight weeks in which to lower their total cholesterol level by diet prior to determining if they were eligible for the study. There is no mention of taking additional steps to secure compliance to dietary recommendations with the help of a dietitian.[14]

The WOSCPS study provided "lipid-lowering dietary advice" at the first screening. Four weeks later the potential subjects were checked again, and if the LDL cholesterol level was over 154 mg/dl (4.0 mmol/l) they were asked to stay on the diet and return in four weeks. Those whose levels were still too high were then randomized. During the trial, dietary advice was "reinforced" during the three-month checkups.[19] Again, who gave the advice and who reinforced it and how, is not reported. One would presume they would mention it if dietitians were assigned this task. As it is, it could have consisted of merely a sentence or two of "reinforcement" by a physician or perhaps a leaflet.

The CARE 1 study offered only four weeks of treatment with the NCEP Step One Diet, and not the recommended six months of intensive dietary therapy, prior to randomization in placebo and drug groups. Patients who still had high LDL cholesterol levels (175 mg/dl or higher) were then put on a Step Two Diet and another cholesterol-lowering drug was also prescribed. No mention is made of involvement of dietitians.[3] Interestingly, despite the fact that the study started in 1989, they refer to the 1993 NCEP guidelines, which are even stricter, as if they followed them. These guidelines require immediate placement of all patients with known heart disease on the Step Two Diet.[28]

In the <u>CARE 2 study</u>, on older men with known heart disease, there is no statement as to how long patients were provided dietary counseling and how intensive it was, only that, "All participants received dietary counseling according to the National Cholesterol Education Program Step 1 guidelines."[20] Given that CARE 2 is only an arbitrarily separated part of the total CARE study, we can assume that these patients were also only provided four weeks of Step One Diet, and not six months of vigorous efforts at treatment by dietary counseling as actually recommended by the NCEP guidelines. They refer to these guidelines but do not provide a reference for them, thus making it difficult for readers to check for themselves and find the discrepancy.

In the <u>Air Force study</u> the minimal Step One dietary measures were started three months in advance and involved three group meetings with a dietitian. After randomization, the participants received "dietary reinforcement" at 12-week intervals, but it is not clear how long this extended.[21] This does not conform to the recommendation of the NCEP which asks for a minimum of six months of intensive dietary therapy and counseling prior to introducing any drug therapy for preventive purposes.

The <u>LIPID study</u> simply did not state which set of dietary guidelines were adopted for its population of patients from Australia and New Zealand, other than that "they received dietary advice aimed at reducing their fat intake to less than 30 percent of total energy intake[24]." This advice was to be followed for eight weeks before the final screening and randomization, and then supported throughout the study. The nature of the advice, who gave it, and its frequency is not mentioned. They did, however, carry out one highly significant action: in order to qualify more participants they prescribed a stricter diet for 700 people who were above the allowable limit for total cholesterol, with the result that 473 of them could then be enrolled.[23] This indicates that they recognized the value of a stricter diet, and that they could get people to follow it.

Recommended Medications: Aspirin and beta blockers

Although aspirin and, to a lesser degree, beta blockers have long been known to effectively lower rates of coronary events for many patients, none of the studies included prescription of these drugs to appropriate patients in either group. We should note here that neither medication would be likely, according to the studies done on these drugs, to lower all-cause mortality.[29,30,31] They would, however, be expected to lower major clinical events and deaths from CHD, which is what all but the 4S study focuses on. Both aspirin and beta blockers are much cheaper than statins: it costs $10,410 to $19,290 to prevent one nonfatal infarction per year with aspirin versus $131,500 to $155,500 with statin drugs.[32,33,34,35]

Proposed Standard V: Use of all-cause and single-cause mortality as the primary end points

The 4S study set as its "primary objective" the reduction of all-cause mortality. Its "secondary objective" was that of the incidence of major cardiovascular disease events, thus lumping together the surrogate end point of nonfatal heart attacks with that of fatal CHD.[14]

None of the other studies set all-cause mortality as a primary end point, at least initially. Presumably, this was because they realized that, given their lower-risk patient populations, they would have to either extend the study longer than the customary five years or increase the number of participants in order to get statistically significant differences. Such extension and enlargement would provide valuable information for physicians and the public, but would be expensive for the pharmaceutical companies.

The LIPID study did an interesting variation on this. In their first paper, they state that the primary objective was to determine the difference in coronary mortality, but that all-cause mortality was also measured in order to "contribute substantially to prospective meta-analyses to detect effects on total mortality."[23] It is as if they did not want to have to stand or fall on this criterion, so they hedged their bets by making it a quasi-primary end point. However, in the study reporting the results, all-cause mortality is given an equal status to that of death from CHD.[24] This promotion may have been prompted by the fact that the difference in all-cause mortality was larger than that of coronary mortality.

The primary end points in the other four studies were deaths from CHD and morbidity from nonfatal myocardial infarction. All-cause mortality was measured but relegated to a secondary status in the WOPCPS and the first CARE study, and was not even reported in the second one. Incidence of stroke was reported across all four studies.

Proposed Standards VI and VII: Measurement of quality of life

None of the studies attempted to measure quality of life, extended or not, much less do a QALY cost analysis.

Proposed Standard VIII: Reporting of differences in risk reduction in absolute terms

The summary of the <u>4S Study</u> reports both relative and absolute risk reductions. That for all-cause mortality was reported as being 12 percent for the controls and eight percent for the drug group — a difference of four percent. However, examination of the tables in the study reveals that 11.5 percent of the controls died within an average of 5.4 years compared to 8.2 percent of the drug group - a 3.3 percent difference. This overall difference was due to the results for men; there was a small difference in the opposite direction with the much smaller group of women in the study.

After this chapter was written the 4S study group reported the results of an additional two years of follow-up.[36] This follow-up showed an increase of difference in all cause survival of 4.4 percent in favor of the drug-taking group, an increase of 1.1 percent over the results at the time of official termination of the study. This increase occurred in spite of the fact that at the termination of the study all subjects were informed of the results to date and were "advised" to take the drug, if they weren't already (not merely informed, but "advised" to do so). This advice apparently was quite effective: 82 percent of the original placebo group reported having switched to statins and 86 percent of the original statin-taking group continued to take the drug. Why then would the original statin group improve on its survival rate in comparison to the placebo group? The authors postulate that it was because it takes a year or two for the drug to start being effective, as indicated by their records during the original study. However, the increase in deaths did not occur primarily because of fewer deaths from coronary causes but for other causes. Only eight of the 23 extra deaths in the original placebo group were due to coronary causes. This suggests other possibilities, namely, that some systematic bias favoring the statin-taking group is at work or that statin drugs have other, unexpected advantages. In any case, the improvement remains in the quite modest range. Further discussion of the 4S study refers to the earlier results at the official termination of the study.[15]

The WOPCPS study reports only relative risk reductions in its summary and in its accounting of "events," coronary and other. Readers must calculate the absolute differences for themselves. This turns out to be an improvement in the survival rate from 95.9 percent for the placebo group to 96.8 percent for the drug group, or less than one percent.[19] It was reported that the difference was nearly statistically significant but it is debatable whether this is of practical significance.

CARE 1 uses both absolute and relative risk reductions in its abstract. However, in its results section all end points were reported only as relative risk reductions. Again, no statistically significant difference was found for all-cause mortality, and the absolute difference was less than one percent.[3]

CARE 2 did not provide data as to all-cause mortality.

Letters to the first three authors (of 13) led to a response from one who provided information about all-cause mortality for the entire CARE study participants. For those less than 65 years of age, there were 88 deaths in the placebo group and 103 in the statin drug group, about a one percent difference in favor of the placebo. This does not correspond with the figures provided by Sacks et al[3] above. Perhaps the change to a one percent advantage for the drug group that CARE 1 reports is due to the inclusion of some patients up to the age of 68. For those 65 and over, there were 108 deaths in the placebo group and 77 in the statin group, an almost five percent difference in favor of the statin group. However, since all-cause mortality was not set up to be a primary end point, statistical significance could not be reliably obtained.[37] Given that the subjects had already suffered a heart attack and were over 70 by the end of the study, it is unlikely that they would live many more years in any case, and the difference between the two groups might well disappear after a couple more years of follow-up.

The AFCAPS/TexCAPS study emphasizes relative risk reductions throughout the article. All-cause mortality is not noted in the section "Efficacy End Points" but instead under the section "Tolerability and Safety." There it can be discovered that there was essentially no difference between the two groups on this measure: 77 total deaths in the placebo group and 80 in the drug group. They found significant differences in nonfatal, single-cause cardiac events but the only other type of morbidity they reported was for cancer, where there were tiny differences in favor of the placebo group for six of the seven types, and a larger difference in favor of the statin group for melanoma.[21,22]

The LIPID study presented the results, in most cases, in both absolute and relative risk reductions, emphasizing the latter in the "Effects on Outcome" section.[24] The difference in favor of the statin group for all-cause mortality (3.1 percent) was actually greater than for death from CHD (1.7 percent).

The following table summarizes the differences between the placebo and the drug groups in the six studies. It includes the category of "Nonfatal Major Coronary Events." This is a surrogate category in terms of determining extension of life since such events may or may not lead to actual death. As noted in chapter three, this may be because such events can act as "wake-up calls" to the victims, and motivate them to institute lifestyle changes. This category is variously defined in the different studies and we have attempted to choose those events that were most consistent in the studies and less apt to overlap with other events. Hence, overt, but not "silent," myocardial infarctions were included, and cardiovascular surgery was not included as this is a treatment, not an original event. The data are consistent with a wake-up call interpretation and evidence of the inadequacy of surrogate categories to predict type and timing of death.

Table 2. **Statin Drug Trials Summary: Differences in absolute percentages (placebo group minus the drug group)**

Study	No. Subjects	Nonfatal Major Coronary Events %	Coronary Mortality %	All-cause Mortality %	Years
4S*	4444	9.0	3.5	3.3	5.4
WOSCPS	6595	1.9	0.7	0.9	4.9
*	4159	0.6	0.9	0.8	5.0
CARE II***	1283	8.4	4.5	4.8	5.0
AFCAPS/ TexCAPS	5608	0.2	0.0	0.0	5.2
LIPID	9014	5.1	1.7	3.1	6.1

* Based on data at termination of study (15)   ** ages 50-68   ***ages 65-75

Proposed Standard IX: Premature termination of study

Both the 4S and the LIPID studies were terminated before their full term at a predetermined statistical level of significance in terms of all-cause mortality. Resultingly, any later diminution or reversal of the targeted benefits of treatment will be difficult or impossible to detect. As noted above, the difference in favor of the drug group was only 3.3 percent in the 4S study and 3.1 percent in the Lipid study.

The AFCAPS/TexCAPS study was programmed to terminate after 320 participants had experienced a primary end point or a minimum after five years after the last participant was randomized, whichever occurred later. Nevertheless, the study was terminated for reasons of "efficacy" after only 267 participants had experienced a primary end point event – first acute major coronary event, unstable angina, or sudden cardiac death. Efficacy was not explained in this context and it seems a rather arbitrary decision, given that there were only eight deaths separating the two groups in terms of all-cause mortality at the end of the study. Since it took almost three years to enroll all the participants, this meant a number of them would not have been followed up for the minimum of five years.

Proposed Standard X: No industry-affiliated ghostwriters

None of the studies indicated whether or not ghostwriters were provided by the pharmaceutical companies funding the study.

Proposed Standard XI: Unbiased publication

Despite the shortcomings in the design of the studies and in the reporting of their results, these studies were nevertheless published in prestigious journals. In most cases the journals also failed to clarify and identify any potential conflicts of interests to the reader. If the journals followed the 1990 AMA guidelines, and apparently only a study published in *JAMA* did[22,] they would have required the clinical investigators involved to disclose "any material ties to companies whose products they are investigating" and been in the position to pass this on to the readers.[38]

Application of Proposed Standards I and II to cost-effectiveness studies

What would be the cost in terms of QALY of prescribing these drugs to all men aged 45 to 64 who have cholesterol levels over 250 mg/dL (6.5mmol/l)? This is difficult to determine for two reasons. The first is that there is no standard way to analyze such data and many, many choices as to how to do it. The second difficulty is that the data with which to make such analyses are incomplete, certainly from the standpoint of the Proposed Standards that would require measurement of quality of life as well as quantity of life. Moreover, the studies did not last long enough to know the eventual outcome for most of the subjects, so that postexperiment costs are basically unknown. We will briefly review three studies that have been done in order to illustrate the problems and the range of conclusions, one on the 4S study, one on the WOSCPS study, and one that looks at populations similar to those of the 4S and WOSCPS participants.

A study that applied the 4S data to Sweden concluded that it would cost $8,968 per discounted life-year gained to take the drug.[39] We won't attempt to explain what "discounted" is other than to say that it is a way of taking into consideration that people are generally more concerned about immediate benefits and costs than long-term ones. The study made several questionable assumptions:

1) The cost of the drug given to the experimental group was only calculated for the 5.4 years of the study, but their estimated additional number of life years varied from 10 to 20, depending on the model. Presumably, they would be taking the drug for at least 10 more years, and, as a result, the total cost per drug taker should be at least three times that which they calculated, or at least $27,000 per life-year gained.

2) The costs were reduced by the amount of fewer expenses for treatment of coronary events in the experimental group than in the placebo group. As pointed out in Proposed Standard II, such "savings" are illusory. Since we all have to die sometime of something, one cannot avoid the costs of illness and death simply by avoiding or postponing treatment of a particular illness.[40,41] Also, since all-cause mortality was only minimally different (3.3 percent) between the two groups in the 4S study, one suspects that the short-term costs accrued from morbidity other than heart disease treatment would largely balance even these "savings."

3) The expenses for the placebo group included a heart transplantation which cost about $93,000. This is an optional procedure, one that is unlikely to meet Proposed Standard I for cost-effectiveness in terms of extended quality of life years gained.

4) They did not include the costs of physician visits and laboratory tests, "as such activities are part of the standard treatment of postmyocardial infarction and angina patients39." This may be true in Sweden but in other countries such standard treatment may be reserved for those who are on drug treatment or have symptoms for which they seek treatment. Also, there are extra tests to determine whether the statin drug is damaging the liver or eyes.

The next study used the WOSCPS data on men without known heart disease but with high cholesterol levels. It determined the cost of life year gained at £20,375 (about $33,000).[25] This included the cost for the Scottish drug patients of monitoring and taking lab tests every six months at about $26 per visit. This is an unrealistically low price by American standards. Otherwise, it made essentially the same questionable assumptions as in the previous study: 1) that the costs occurred for treatment of fewer coronary events should be subtracted; 2) that only costs for the first five years of drugs should be included, whereas there is no reason to believe that the patients would not take them indefinitely; and 3) that the patients, albeit with presumably unhealthily high levels of cholesterol, would live out a normal life span (average of 15 more years). Points 2 and 3 were noted by writers of letters to the editor.[42,43] Without these assumptions the cost per life year gained would be £89,000 ($145,000), or almost three times as much.

The third study, carried out by Pharoah and Hollingworth[44], projected the data from both the 4S study and the WOSCPS study onto a population in a typical district health authority in England. It reports:

The average cost-effectiveness for treating men aged 45-64 with no history of coronary heart disease and a cholesterol concentration of 6.5 mmol/l [251mg/dL] and higher for 10 years with a statin was £136,000 [$221,680] per life year saved. The average cost effectiveness for patients with pre-existing coronary heart disease and a cholesterol concentration greater than 5.5 mmol/l [212 mg/dL] was £32,000 [$52,160].

What a difference a few assumptions make: from $8,968 per life year gained to $52,160 for men with known heart disease, or almost six times as much, and from $33,211 to $221,680 for men without known heart disease but with high cholesterol! How is this possible? The main reason is that Pharoah and Hollingworth[44], contrary to the previous studies[25,39], extended the cost of the drugs for ten years. Another reason is that the cholesterol levels of the men in the group that they used without known heart disease were slightly lower than those of the participants in the WOSCPS trial. This put them at a lower risk of CHD which has the effect of increasing the cost of achieving the same amount of life extension.

Even at that, Pharoah and Hollingworth[44] were conservative in their estimates in that they did not include office visits or other costs associated with the drug treatment and, similar to the other two studies, they included the "savings" from less treatment for coronary events. Thus, even their costs were an underestimate.

A simpler way to estimate the cost of a treatment is exemplified by an American physician in a letter to the editor. It is not only so simple that almost anyone can apply it but it also has the advantage of being accurate in terms of the local price of the product or procedure.[45] The physician used the data from the WOSCPS study and applied it to his practice. All he needed was the cost of the drug per month and the number of high-risk patients who had to be treated to postpone one death. He could obtain the first figure from his practice and the last figure by finding the absolute difference between the drug and the placebo groups in terms of the end point in which he was interested. In the case of death from CHD, the difference was 0.07 percent. Dividing that into 100 he calculated that 143 patients would have to be treated for one death to be postponed past five years. He then multiplied the drug cost per month ($100) by the number of months the study lasted (60). **He multiplied this number ($6,000) by 143 and determined that it would cost $858,000 to postpone one death past five years. For women this figure would exceed $3.4 million** because of the lower rate of development of CHD in women. These costs would be less in Europe and Canada as the statin drugs cost less there, but can be computed using the same formula.

SUMMARY OF APPLICATION OF THE RELEVANT PROPOSED STANDARDS TO THE COST-ANALYSIS STUDIES

Proposed Standards I and 11: Cost-analysis

All three articles violated the gold standards on costs. The cost of the drug treatment, once corrected for obviously faulty assumptions, probably easily exceeded the average, annual total expenditures of a single-parent, single-child family in the countries in which the statin drugs were most apt to be used ($22,626 in 1995 in the USA). Also, they included as "savings" costs that are merely postponed rather than eliminated. This would have raised the cost of treatment even more.

Proposed Standard III: Disclosure of Conflict of Interest

The original cost-analysis study that applied the 4S study results to Sweden did not report its source of funding.[39] This was not required in the European journal in which it was first published. It does, though, list an employee of the drug company among its list of participating investigators. Essentially the same study was also published later in the *New England Journal of Medicine* where it was stated that the drug manufacturer funded the study.[46]

The cost-analysis study that applied the WOSCPS study results to Britain was paid for by the drug company which sold the drug.[25] Several members of the analysis group, including the head of the executive committee, also received money from the company for other work. This same person was one of the investigator-authors who produced the original study.

In stark contrast, the Pharoah and Hollingworth[44] study, which made the most objective analysis, states clearly at the end of the paper, and in the same sized print: "Funding: None. Conflict of interest: None."

Proposals for Reducing/Eliminating Conflicts of Interest

Other statin trials are in progress. However, the "successful" mold has been established and it is doubtful whether that they will depart much from it. It will be unlikely that these studies will take on real tiger opponents, such as comparing statins to strict, strongly supported dietary measures (which were cited earlier); all-cause mortality will remain unpopular as a primary end point; measurement of all-cause reported treatment to be used in QALY analysis of cost and quality of life will not be done; truly long-term studies to see what actually happens over 10 or 15 years to the participants will be rare or nonexistent; and there will be no strict regulation of conflict of interest of the principals involved

One way in which to make drug studies more credible would be for governments to pay the members of an independent oversight committee and insure that none of them are connected to the drug company. At the minimum, this committee's duties would be to receive all data, determine their independent validity and accuracy, and conduct all analyses of them. It would make an independent, publicly available, report to the government of its findings. In the USA, funds for such committees could come from the reduction of the tax exemptions provided to pharmaceutical companies.

This would be a partial safeguard. It would not do much, if anything, towards designing studies in such a way as to test drugs against other than "straw men" conditions.

A more far-reaching change would require drug companies to pay into a common fund which would then be used to carry out the required clinical studies. The drug companies would not have any say over the design of the projects, nor do any of the analysis of the data, nor provide any assistance in writing up or otherwise presenting any of the results, nor have any prepublication rights to review and comment on any presentations or proposed publications prior to their occurrence. And they certainly would not be able to hire any of the people working on such research or otherwise reward them during or soon after such research projects were finished. Nor would these people or their family members be allowed to invest money in such businesses.

Such a model could apply to other commercial interests that need clinical trials to get approval of their products or procedures. It would be interesting to see what results would be obtained. It would have the advantage for commercial interests that whatever products or procedures survived such a process would be more trustworthy. But without the application of the Proposed Standards to all the research projects, independently done or not, real trust would not be warranted. The investigators involved, for example, will still be interested in publication and, unless journal editors removed publication biases in favor of "positive results," the incentive will be to continue to set up straw men comparisons.

References

[1] Pope, Alexander (1688-1744). English poet and satirist. Excerpt from his *"Letter to Fortescue,"* dated September 23, 1725.

[2] Hulley SB, Newman TB, et al. (1993). Should we be measuring blood cholesterol levels in young adults? *JAMA* 269: 1416-19.

[3] Sacks FM, Pfeffer MA, et al. (1996). The effect of pravastatin on coronary events after myocardial infarction in patients with average cholesterol levels. *N Engl J Med* 335: 1001-09.

[4] Wald NJ, Law M, et al. (1994). Aplipoproteins and ischaemic heart disease: implications for screening. *Lancet* 343: 75-79.

[5] Henderson A (1996). Coronary heart disease: overview. *Lancet* 348: s1-s4.

[6] De Lorgeril M, Salen P, et al. (1999). Mediterranean diet, traditional risk factors, and the rate of cardiovascular complications after myocardial infarction. Final report of the Lyons Diet Heart Study. *Circulation* 99: 779-85.

[7] GISSI-Prevenzione Investigators (1999). Dietary supplementation with n-3 polyunsaturated fatty acids and vitamin E after myocardial infarction: results of the GISSI-Prevenzione trial. *Lancet* 354: 447-55.

[8] Temple NJ (1996). Dietary fats and coronary heart disease. *Biomedicine Pharmacotherapy* 50: 261-68.

[9] Singh RB, Rastogi SS, et al. (1992). Randomized controlled trial of cardioprotective diet in patients with recent acute myocardial infarction: Results of one year follow up. *BMJ* 304: 1015-19.

[10] Ornish D, Scherwitz LW, et al. (1998). Intensive lifestyle changes for reversal of coronary heart disease. *JAMA* 280: 2001-07.

[11] Muldoon MF, Criqui MH (1997). The emerging role of statins in the prevention of coronary heart disease. *BMJ* 315: 1554-55.

[12] Ebrahim S, Smith GD, et al. (1998). Cholesterol and coronary heart disease: screening and treatment. *Quality Health Care* 7: 232-39.

[13] CQ Staff (February 7, 1998). How each agency and department would fare under Clinton budget. *Congressional Quarterly* 297-314.

[14] Scandinavian Simvastatin Survival Study Group (1993). Design and baseline results of the Scandinavian Simvastatin Survival Study of patients with stable angina and/or previous myocardial infarction. *Am J Cardiol* 71: 393-99.

[15] Scandinavian Simvastatin Survival Study Group (1994). Randomized trial of cholesterol lowering in 4444 patients with coronary heart disease: the Scandinavian Simvastatin Survival Study. *Lancet* 344: 1383-89.

[16] Schultz KF, Chalmers I et al. (1995). Empirical evidence of bias. *JAMA* 273: 408-12.

[17] Ravnskov U (1992). Cholesterol lowering trials in coronary heart disease: frequency of citation and outcome. *BMJ* 305: 15-19.

[18] The West of Scotland Coronary Prevention Study Group (1992). A coronary primary prevention study of Scottish men aged 45-64: Trial design. *J Clin Epidemiol* 45: 849-60.

[19] Shepherd J, Cobbe SM, et al. (1995). Prevention of coronary heart disease with pravastatin in men with hypercholesterolemia. *N Engl J Med* 333: 1301-07.

[20] Lewis SJ, Moye LA, et al. (1998). Effect of Pravastatin on cardiovascular events in older patients with myocardial infarction and cholesterol levels in the average range. *Ann Intern Med* 129: 681-89.

[21] Downs JR, Beere PA, et al. (1997). Design percent rational of the Air Force/Texas Coronary Atherosclerosis Prevention Study. *Am J Cardiol* 80: 287-93.

[22] Downs JR, Clearfield M, et al. (1998). Primary prevention of acute coronary events with Lovastatin in men and women with average cholesterol levels. *JAMA* 279: 1615-22.

[23] The LIPID Study Group (1995). Design features and baseline characteristics of the LIPID (Long-Term Intervention with Pravastatin in Ischemic Disease) study. *Am J Cardiol* 76: 474-79.

[24] The Long-Term Intervention with Pravastatin in Ischemic Disease Study Group (1998). *N Engl J Med* 339: 1349-57.

[25] Caro J, Klittich W, et al. (1997). The West of Scotland Prevention Study: economic benefit analysis of primary prevention with pravastatin. *BMJ* 315: 1577-82.

[26] Study Group, European Atherosclerosis Society (1987). Strategies for the prevention of coronary heart disease: a policy statement of the European Atherosclerosis Society. *Eur Heart J* 8: 77-88.

[27] Expert Panel (1988). Report of the National Cholesterol Education Program Expert Panel on detection, evaluation, and treatment of high blood cholesterol in adults. *Arch Intern Med* 148: 36-60.

[28] Expert panel on detection, evaluation, and treatment of high blood cholesterol in adults (1993). Summary of the Second Report of the National Cholesterol Education Program (NCEP) Expert Panel on Detection, Evaluation, and Treatment of High Blood Cholesterol in Adults (Adult Treatment Panel II). *JAMA* 269: 3015-23.

[29] Antiplatelet trialists collaboration (1998). Secondary prevention of vascular disease by prolonged antiplatelet treatment. *BMJ* 296: 320-31.

[30] Glynn R J, Buring J E, et al. (1994). Adherence to aspirin in the prevention of myocardial infarction. *Arch Intern Med* 154: 2649-57.

[31] Verheught FWA (1998). Aspirin, the poor man's statin. *Lancet* 351: 227-28.

[32] Horton R (1994). Reversing risk in coronary disease *Lancet* 344: 1497-98.

[33] Kmietowicz Z (1998). Aspirin and warfarin best for primary prevention of heart attacks. *BMJ* 316: 330.

[34] Marwick C (1997). Aspirin's role in prevention now official. *JAMA* 277: 701-02.

[35] Sharpe N (1999). Benefit of beta blockers for heart failure: proven in 1999. *Lancet* 353: 1988-89.

[36] Pedersen TR, Wilhelmsen L, et al. (2000). Follow-up study of patients randomized in the Scandinavian Simvastatin Survival Study (4S) of cholesterol lowering. *Amer J Cardiol* 86: 257-262.

[37] Moye L (October 25 and 27, 1999). Personal communication.

[38] Council on Scientific Affairs and Council on Ethical and Judicial Affairs (1990). Conflicts of interest in medical center/industry research relationships. *JAMA* 263: 2790-93.

[39] Jönsson B, Johannesson M, et al. (1996). Cost effectiveness of cholesterol lowering. *Eur Heart J* 17: 1101-07.

[40] St. Leger, HS (1998). Earlier study of effect on healthcare costs of preventing fatal diseases yielded similar results. *BMJ* 316: 1985.

[41] Bonneux L, Barendregt JJ, et al. (1998). Preventing fatal diseases increase healthcare costs: cause elimination life table approach. *BMJ* 316: 26-29.

[42] Pharoah P (1998). Modeling economic benefits after such long-term treatment is inappropriate. *BMJ* 316: 1241.

[43] Freemantle N, Mason J (1998). Assumptions are methodologically flawed. *BMJ* 316: 1241.

[44] Pharoah PDP, Hollingworth W (1996). Cost effectiveness of lowering cholesterol concentration with statins in patients with and without pre-existing coronary heart disease. *BMJ* 312: 1443-48.

[45] Rogers S (1996). Prevention of coronary heart disease with pravastatin. *N Engl J Med* 334: 1333.

[46] Johannesson M, Jönsson B, et al. (1997). Cost effectiveness of simvastatin treatment to lower cholesterol levels in patients with coronary heart disease. *N Engl J Med* 336: 332-36.

Chapter Eight

The Right Heart Catheter: Evidence versus Bias
Stephen Workman

Critically ill patients are worrisome for physicians. Threatening imminent death, they often defy complete understanding. In developed nations most such patients are managed in the intensive care unit (ICU) where they frequently receive a right heart catheter (RHC) (also known as a Swan Ganz catheter or a pulmonary artery catheter (PAC)). This is a monitoring device inserted into the heart. Developed in the 1940s, the RHC is now used in the ICU to monitor the function of the heart, providing information that allows the generation of data useful to assist in therapeutic efforts to improve the function of the heart. The "swan" as it has come to be referred to by those who use it, and the data it can be used to generate has become an integral part of caring for critically ill patients. While the RHC was initially only used in cardiac laboratories, it was adopted in the ICU after an article published in 1970 demonstrated an effective "bedside" technique for its insertion and use.[1]

The following case description conveys why the RHC has become integral to the care of critically ill patients. While working as an internist covering the emergency room in a secondary-care hospital, a 74-year-old man was urgently referred to me. Despite having a blood pressure much less than normal he had managed to walk into the emergency department. He was, however, confused, as the blood supply to his brain was already severely compromised. He appeared ashen and unwell, soaked with sweat, and had the peculiar odor that individuals in shock develop. Had he been unhealthy with narrowed blood vessels in his brain or heart he would have already been unconscious, with an expected mortality rate of over 80 percent.[2] In an attempt to perfuse vital organs — the heart, brain, and kidneys — his body had already shunted blood away from nonessential tissues. His arms and legs were bluish, clammy and cold and mottled, and his skin was pale. He had no clear evidence as to the cause of his illness.

Laboratory tests showed his body was starved of blood and oxygen, and it was likely he would die shortly if a diagnosis were not reached and

117

A. Thompson and N.J. Temple (eds.), Ethics, Medical Research, and Medicine, 117–128.
© 2001 *Kluwer Academic Publishers. Printed in the Netherlands.*

treatments started soon. He had only a modestly increased white blood cell count, and slightly impaired function of the kidneys suggesting he was at risk of proceeding to "multisystem failure." Left untreated his disease would progress, and organ systems, would, one by one, begin to fail. Gut, lungs, kidneys, brain, bone marrow, liver, like dominoes tumbling in a row, each would bow out in turn. Within 24 hours the patient could be reduced to little more than a large collection of cells, cells devoted, not to maintaining organ function, but instead devoted only to staying alive. When multisystem failure develops, patients face mortality rates from 50 to 90 percent. Those who survive can require treatment in an ICU for weeks or months, often unresponsive for much of this time. Such outcomes are horrific for patients, their family members, and for the ICU staff who must care for them. In some cases the patient does not die from the disease directly, but remains in limbo, dying only after the deliberate withdrawal of life-sustaining treatments, an often agonizing and heart-rending process. In short, things could go very, very badly.

If the patient was in shock due to an overwhelming infection, known as septic shock, then his heart was starved for blood, the arteries and veins in his body dilated in response to the infection, pooling blood before it reached the heart. If septic, he would need intravenous fluids, sometimes ten or more liters. Unfortunately, if he were in shock due to a problem with his heart, as happens to patients with a heart attack, intravenous fluids could flood into his lungs causing respiratory failure, further threatening his life.

Fortunately, the RHC offered a way out from this dilemma. The RHC is a meter-long flexible tube approximately 3mm in diameter. The end of the catheter contains a tiny balloon that can be inflated to guide it through the blood vessels. It is inserted into a large vein in the neck and travels to the heart, then into a blood vessel leading into the lungs.

By measuring pressures and determining the pumping capacity of the heart, the RHC provides information that allowed me to understand and quantify the function of the heart. The information indicated that the patient's left heart was not receiving enough blood and that the man was, in fact, in septic shock. He was given many liters of intravenous fluid and showed some improvement. But when this did not adequately improve the numbers, the RHC also guided the administration of adrenaline like drugs to increase the blood pressure. Through the use of the RHC, diagnostic certainty was obtained, and a variety of "secondary" endpoints, such as blood pressure, oxygen delivery, and cardiac output, were improved. The patient turned out to have a rare but devastating and rapidly progressive bacterial infection. Within 24 hours his condition had improved significantly, and ten days later he walked out of the hospital. Clearly, the RHC played an important role in ensuring the patient's survival.

HISTORY OF THE RHC

The first scientific report describing the bedside use of the "swan ganz" catheter, named after its inventors, Drs Swan and Ganz, was published in the prestigious *New England Journal of Medicine* in 1970.[1] The article described the rationale for the catheter's use, along with the technique required to insert it without use of X-ray equipment to ensure correct placement. The paper did not present data showing an improvement in survival. The device was not required to undergo testing by the Food and Drug Administration before being licensed for use, and, for over 20 years few clinical trials were conducted to examine the efficacy of the catheter in the treatment of critically ill patients. However, perhaps due to the clear utility of the RHC in obtaining secondary endpoints such as blood pressure and oxygen delivery, physicians easily and intuitively accepted the usefulness of the device. Currently, it is estimated that 1.5 million RHCs are used each year in the United States.

Some risks were appreciated quite early on. Since the inserting a RHC requires "blindly" penetrating the body with a large needle, and then inserting a foreign object through the needle and into the heart and blood vessels, complications were not unexpected. That the catheter can be harmful was driven home to me in 1997 when, purely by chance, I happened across a 25-year-old magazine, wedged behind the seat of a subway car. The article described a previously healthy university student who suffered severe brain damage after physicians had inserted a RHC as part of a research experiment. The tip of the catheter passing through the heart caused a cardiac arrest. The student suffered severe brain injury before heart function could be restored. The medical literature also clearly describes the many other risks of inserting a RHC. A medline® search for articles containing the word "swan-ganz" in the title published since 1970 returned 433 articles. Of these 163 were case reports or series or articles devoted to describing complications associated with the catheter. Indeed, the first medline® article containing the word "swan-ganz" is entitled: "Perforation of the pulmonary artery by a Swan-Ganz catheter."[3]

Other complications included bleeding around the puncture site, stroke, loss of the catheter into the body, knotting of the catheter precluding removal, puncture of the heart resulting in a potentially lethal accumulation of blood around the heart, heart attacks, "balloon rupture" of the pulmonary artery causing bleeding into the lungs, arrhythmias (both fatal and benign), introduction of air into the bloodstream or the chest cavity, penetration of the catheter into the space around the spinal cord, infection of the catheter or the valves of the heart, damage to the heart valves from the catheter, clotting of blood vessels, and suturing of the catheter to the heart muscle during operations. These "mechanical" complications have become an unwanted, but acceptable side effect of the use of the RHC.

Such anecdotal evidence of complications are, of course, easily discounted since they present only the risks and offer no statistical measure of effectiveness. Consequently, knowledge of the "mechanical" complications did not and has not deterred physicians from utilizing the catheter widely for over 30 years. The widespread acceptance of the RHC, despite the obvious risks, likely arose for a variety of reasons, some of which are apparent in the illustrative case. First, many very sick patients die in the ICU. Doing nothing is not an appealing option.[4,5] Severe illnesses require what is commonly referred to as "aggressive treatment." Potential complications from such treatment are likely to be acceptable. Second, since "mechanical" complications occur in only 0.1 to 0.5% of patients[6,7], they are unlikely to occur repetitively to any particular physician or in any ICU. Third, the capacity to solve the mechanical complications that can arise during the use of a RHC is well developed. Numerous papers have been published describing techniques to remove a "knotted" RHC. Fourth, doing nothing requires acknowledging some level of helplessness in an ICU environment, an environment designed for intervention and activity. (In presenting the mindset for **not** using the RHC one author stated: "Don't just do something, stand there."[8] Fifth, the RHC offers both ritual and reassurance to the physician. The patient is covered in a large sterile blue sheet, while the physician is gowned and gloved, perhaps anxious to reduce a mysterious and dangerous disease to a collection of easily manipulated numeric data. The ability to manipulate numeric data creates a sense of control that is reassuring. Sixth, inserting a RHC offers tangible evidence to patients and family members, as well as one's peers, that one is doing "everything." Indeed, once RHCs are widely adopted, failure to use one suggests that one is not practicing within the legal and ethical "standard of care." In litigious societies this gives rise to the fear of a malpractice lawsuit. Seventh, RHCs allow physicians to pursue and attain secondary endpoints, such as blood pressure and cardiac output, that are easily perceived as therapeutic. Finally, there is an economic incentive to use a RHC. While working as an internist, I would receive $100 (US) for every consult I saw after midnight, but would be paid $175 for inserting a RHC, a procedure which in skilled hands takes less time. I would also receive another $40 to $80 per day while the RHC was in place.

In short, many years after the widespread adoption of the RHC there were many substantive reasons and pressures for physicians to routinely use the RHC, and only anecdotal evidence against their use.

RECENT RESEARCH ON THE RHC

A large study (the SUPPORT Study) of 5,700 critically ill patients found that those on whom the RHC was used had a significantly higher rate of mortality than those not administered the RHC.[9] Only 46 percent of those given the RHC survived six months versus 54 percent who did not receive the RHC. This difference was highly statistically significant and of obvious clinical importance. When the 1,008 RHC recipients were matched in disease category and appropriateness for its use to 1,008 nonrecipients, the difference between the two groups in probability of survival was reduced from eight percent to five percent, still of both practical and statistical significance. Further analysis, based upon diagnostic groupings, did not reveal any disease process, such as septic or cardiogenic shock, that benefited from the use of a RHC. The bill for the RHC recipients was $13,600 more than those for their matched pairs.

Since the assignment of the RHC was done by physician judgment, this type of study is called an "observational study." The alternative study design is an experimental one in which the assignment is done randomly. That type of study design is supposed to reduce biases. This was compensated for in the study by matching the patients and by statistical adjustments of important variables, with the result that the study is the next best thing to a randomly controlled trial. It provides by far the best evidence to date concerning the value of the RHC as a diagnostic intervention.

Despite the strength of the findings and the exhaustive efforts taken to adjust for confounding variables, the authors of the study were somewhat equivocal in their conclusions. Discounting their own findings, the authors were unwilling to conclude that the use of the RHC was, in fact, harmful to the critically ill patients they studied. An accompanying editorial displayed a similar reluctance to accept the data. This editorial was entitled: "Is it time to pull the Pulmonary Artery Catheter?"[10] (Perhaps the first two words in the title should have been reversed.) The authors of the editorial suggested a moratorium, but then stated that they would "greatly prefer a randomized trial to a moratorium."

Despite conclusions that were softer than the data, criticism was immediate. There were several common arguments and responses against the study results. It was argued that patients received a RHC because they were recognized by their physicians to be at greater risk of dying.[11] This explanation cannot, however, explain the increase in mortality being spread throughout the different prognostic groups, and was also explicitly addressed by carefully controlling for prognostic variables in the data analysis. Indeed, if there were an unidentified variable in the prognostic model that accounted for the increase in mortality rate in those patients who received a RHC, the unidentified variable would have been larger than the top six predictive variables. Nonetheless, from my discussions with ICU physicians, the observational design of the study is the most common reason given for discounting the results. A recent review study has shown that observational studies can provide the same results as randomized and controlled studies.[12,13] Good evidence comes from good studies, which have as much to do with execution as design.

Another common response to the results was: "Yes, in the wrong hands the RHC is dangerous, but I know of patients who have benefited from its use." Indeed, a variation of this claim was made in a letter by one of the authors of the original editorial that called for a moratorium on the use of RHC, who stated that he was aware of patients whose condition was improved through the use of the RHC. Claims of efficacy based upon variation in skill levels disregard the "real world" design of the study, which was conducted in teaching hospitals, commonly considered centers of excellence. It is also, of course, impossible for all patients to receive care only from those with the greatest expertise.

A third argument against the results is that there is no clear causal mechanism to explain the increase in mortality.[14] There is an association but no mechanistic explanation and therefore the results of the study are supposedly not compelling. Tobacco companies used this argument for years, saying that since there was no known mechanism by which smoking has been shown to cause cancer, there was only an association, but no direct evidence of causation. The great majority of physicians never accepted this argument. A lack of known mechanism is not surprising in the case of the RHC. Since very little is known about the process of multisystem failure, and there is no effective treatment for it beyond supportive care, it is not surprising that the mechanism by which RHCs increase mortality remains unknown.

While many argued vociferously against the results, other responses were, at least on the surface, more accepting. One common response was to call for a randomized controlled study, a "gold standard" study, to resolve the controversy.

The intense criticism of the study appeared to be heeded. The authors of the editorial that went so far as to demand a moratorium if a controlled trial was not undertaken, further softened their position in response to the letters. One stated: "I am an advocate of the catheter and have used it extensively. Although I cannot prove it, I think there are subgroups of patients in whom the PA catheter has improved survival." The other author noted that the "hard line" position of a moratorium was in fact intended to "stimulate the National Heart Lung and Blood Institute to undertake an appropriate randomized clinical trial."

The economic costs of continuing to use the RHC were never mentioned during the debate or in the article. A 1997 article looking at the cost effectiveness of the RHC did not base a cost-effectiveness analysis upon the SUPPORT study data, but instead concluded that "economic analyses and cost effectiveness are moot prior to the establishment of clinical efficacy....until the clinical questions are answered."[15]

The SUPPORT study does demonstrate that the cost of the widespread usage of the RHC is in the billions of dollars. According to the manufacturers, over 1.5 million are used in the USA annually[16], at an estimated direct cost of over two billion dollars per year.[15] The additional costs of using RHCs must also be considerable. The SUPPORT study showed that use of a RHC was associated with an average cost increase of $14,000 per patient, an increase in costs of almost 40 percent. Since ICU expenditures in the United States consume one percent of the GDP, approximately 80 billion dollars, and 10 percent of patients in the ICU receive a RHC, the additional costs would also be measured in billions of dollars. Calls to address the financial incentives for physicians or hospitals to utilize RHCs have not been advanced.

The problem of "competing interests" and the use of the RHC was never raised during the debate following the publication of the SUPPORT study. (A representative of The American College of Cardiology, a group of physicians who frequently utilize the RHC, stated in a letter that due to under-representation of patients with acute heart attacks in the study, the findings should not be applied to their patients.[17] In a letter of response, the lead author of the SUPPORT study agreed with this criticism, not mentioning the four previous observational studies cited in the SUPPORT study,[18,19,20,21] all of which demonstrated that patients suffering heart attacks who received a RHC had an increased mortality rate.

One solution would be to remove RHCs from fee schedules for the treatment of critically ill patients since they are at best unproven treatment. The question for third party payers is clear: Why pay for treatments that the best available evidence suggests increase costs and don't work?

PROBLEMS IN INVESTIGATING TREATMENTS

The failure of the RHC to improve outcomes together with the difficulty in limiting usage of a widely accepted treatment is also seen in other studies that challenge current treatment practices. Often secondary end points are used to justify a treatment rather than hard end points, such as death. In 1998, the commonly accepted practice of giving critically ill patients albumin, a human protein extracted from blood, was shown to be harmful, increasing the absolute risk of a patient dying by six percent when compared to intravenous saline.[22] The study combined 30 older randomized trials in order to obtain a significant result. The accompanying editorial stated that: "The administration of albumin should be halted until, as the authors suggest, the results of a high quality large clinical trial are available."[23] Similar to the SUPPORT study response, this position was modified by the author on the journal website on the day of publication. "Halted" the author explained, actually meant "....clinicians should pause and consider the issues of validity, clinical relevance, and applicability as presented in the editorial before giving albumin to the next critically ill patient."[24] The majority of letters to the editor were again critical of the article's conclusions. Indeed, the arguments supporting the use of albumin were similar to those in favor of the use of the RHC: inadequacy of research techniques, it was not a randomized trial and the findings are therefore not definitive, theoretical advantages for the use of albumin, and under-representation of particular patient groups. The authors of the article however noted that correspondents did not provide any evidence that albumin is beneficial for critically ill patients. In contrast to the debate about the RHC, the issue of competing interests was raised. One author described an offer by the manufacturers of albumin to pay for him to attend a conference in California examining the use of albumin. He was offered $1500 US to cover ancillary expenses.

Other common practices have also recently been challenged. A recent analysis of the effectiveness of feeding of critically ill patients intravenously failed to show any clear benefits and demonstrated that the practice was harmful to very ill patients.[25] Similarly, a recent study showed that giving blood transfusions intended to maintain a more normal hemoglobin level doubled the mortality rate for the less sick patients, from 8 to 16 percent, and increased mortality from 18 to 23 percent in the sicker patients.[26] (The second increase in mortality was not statistically significant.)

There are several lessons to be learned from these studies, as well as the reactions of the medical establishment to them. First, making numbers better, or pursuing secondary end points, is not synonymous with making patients better. RHCs improve cardiac outputs, blood transfusions improve hemoglobin levels, and albumin decreases edema and improves the measured serum albumin. The end point improves while the patient worsens.

The potential for secondary end points to generate misleading findings was clearly demonstrated in the following study. It was believed that drugs which suppress extra heartbeats (premature ventricular contractions, or PVCs) in-patients with heart disease could prevent them from dying from a sustained run of extra beats called ventricular tachycardia, a common cause of sudden death. The "PVC" suppression trial, called the CAST, trial clearly showed that while the drugs prevent PVCs, they also increase the likelihood of the patient dying.[27] Since the results were based upon a randomized controlled trial, they were widely accepted.

As the easy acceptance of the CAST trial demonstrated, evidence based medicine is a double-edged sword that "cuts both ways." Since "evidence" in evidence based medicine has become synonymous with randomized, double-blinded, and ideally, placebo-controlled trials, it is easy for clinicians to disregard the results of observational studies if they conflict with current treatment practices. For example, in a debate with the author of the SUPPORT study, the president of the American Society of Critical Care stated, "In the absence of randomized controlled trials, it is impossible to say whether RHCs are overused, or what their effect is on mortality....Connors et al. did a good retrospective study. Such studies raise questions that can best be answered by prospective ones."[28] A recent report from a recent multi-author workshop that examined the use of the RHC also discounted the possibility of harm.[16] It stated that: "A recent ...study raised perhaps the greatest concern, potential harm associated with PAC use." In fact, the results of the study did not suggest that "potential harm" was associated with PAC use, they clearly showed that harm was associated. Besides the obvious explanation, namely that the results are in fact correct, the only other possible explanation for the association is that of a flawed study. The authors continued, "Some large observational studies have even suggested that excess morbidity and mortality are associated with the use of the PAC." (Emphasis added; no references were provided.) The authors then noted that: "an actual cause and effect relationship has not been established" due to a lack of adequately powered randomized and controlled trials. Such evidence bias makes it especially difficult to address unproven but widely accepted treatments. A randomized Canadian trial intended to determine the usefulness of the RHC did not advance because many physicians would not enroll patients in the study, believing it would be unethical not to provide such a widely accepted treatment.

Another lesson to be learned is that the mechanism of action of a treatment and the intuitive rationale behind it contribute to the reluctance of physicians to abandon it. Right heart catheters, unlike drugs, are used differently by different physicians, and are perceived as being highly "operator dependent." This source of variability can easily result in physicians viewing the effectiveness of the RHC as a measure of their effectiveness and competence. Individual variability also allows individual physicians to claim that negative outcome data should not be applied to them. (A key problem with this position is that, even if the treatments were shown to be effective and improved the relative likelihood of survival by five percent or so, such an improvement would be well below the limit of that which a perceptive physician could discern at the bedside.)

A reluctance or unwillingness to simultaneously examine both costs and efficacy is another problem as this separation results in two different standards of cost effectiveness, one for proven treatments, another for "unproven" treatments. This separations allows supporters of unproven but likely ineffective treatments, such as the RHC, to ignore costs until efficacy is known for certain. A reluctance to undertake clinical trials that are likely, if anything, to substantially decrease the income of the involved physicians is not surprising.

This problem of competing interests makes it difficult for physicians to even talk openly about the cost of treatment. I had the opportunity to meet the head investigator of the SUPPORT study, Dr Alfred Connors, a man of Lincolnesque bearing and proportion. He had presented the results of the study earlier in the day to a group of intensive care physicians, and I went out for lunch with him and a half dozen or so of the intensive care physicians. I was the only nonintensivist present at the table. I remember feeling that I was the only person really interested in continuing to talk about the results of the study.

"Well, what about the financial incentive to use a Swan Ganz? To what extent does that drive their use? They must generate a lot of income for hospitals and physicians. Has the amount ever been quantified?" I somewhat blithely asked. My question was followed by what I remember to be an extremely clear and distinct silence. Conversation around the table halted. I felt very uncomfortable, and waited with bated breath. There was a pause while Dr Connors carefully composed his answer. "No. I don't think cost is a consideration," he said. Point dismissed. After another pause, a pause during which everyone took a few seconds to relax, conversation resumed.

References

[1] Swan HJ, Ganz W, et al. (1970). Catheterization of the heart in man with use of a flow-directed balloon-tipped catheter. *N Engl J Med* 283: 447-51.

[2] Leibovici L, Drucker M, et al. (1997). Septic shock in bacteremic patients: risk factors, features and prognosis. *Scand J Infect Dis* 29: 71-75.

[3] Chun GM, Ellestad MH. (1971). Perforation of the pulmonary artery by a Swan-Ganz catheter. *N Engl J Med* 284: 1041-42.

[4] Mahul P, Perrot D, et al. (1991). Short- and long-term prognosis, functional outcome following ICU for elderly. *Intensive Care Med* 17: 7-10.

[5] Rauss A, Knaus WA. et al. (1990). Prognosis for recovery from multiple organ system failure: the accuracy of objective estimates of *chances for survival. The French Multicentric Group of ICU Research. Med Decis Making* 10: 155-62.

[6] Hogue CW, Jr., Lappas GD, et al. (1995). Swallowing dysfunction after cardiac operations. Associated adverse outcomes and risk factors including intraoperative transesophageal echocardiography. *J Thorac Cardiovasc Surg* 110: 517-22.

[7] Tuman KJ, McCarthy RJ, et al. (1989). Effect of pulmonary artery catheterization on outcome in patients undergoing coronary artery surgery. *Anesthesiology* 70: 199-206.

[8] Hall JB. (2000). Use of the pulmonary artery catheter in critically ill patients: was invention the mother of necessity? *JAMA* 283: 2577-78.

[9] Connors AF, Speroff T, et al. (1996). The effectiveness of right heart catheterization in the initial care of critically ill patients. SUPPORT Investigators. *JAMA* 276: 889-97.

[10] Dalen JE, Bone RC. (1996). Is it time to pull the pulmonary artery catheter? *JAMA* 276: 916-18.

[11] Baxter JK, Beilman GJ, Abrams JH. (1997). Effectiveness of right heart catheterization: time for a randomized trial. *JAMA* 277: 108.

[12] Concato J. Shah N, Horwitz RI. (2000). Randomized, controlled trials, observational studies, and the hierarchy of research designs. *N Engl J Med* 342: 1887-92.

[13] Benson K, Hartz AJ. (2000). A comparison of observational studies and randomized, controlled trials. *N Engl J Med* 342: 1878-86.

[14] Heyland D, Aitken S, Drover J. (1997). Effectiveness of right heart catheterization: time for a randomized trial. *JAMA* 277:110.

[15] Chalfin DB. (1997). The pulmonary artery catheter: economic aspects. *New Horiz* 5: 292-96.

[16] Bernard GR, Sopko G, et al. (2000). Pulmonary artery catheterization and clinical outcomes: National Heart, Lung, and Blood Institute and Food and Drug Administration Workshop Report. Consensus Statement. *JAMA* 283: 2568-72.

[17] Lewis RP. (1997). Effectiveness of right heart catheterization: time for a randomized trial. *JAMA* 277: 109.

[18] Gore JM, Goldberg RJ, et al. (1987). A community-wide assessment of the use of pulmonary artery catheters in patients with acute myocardial infarction. *Chest* 92: 721-27.

[19] Zion MM, Balkin J, et al. (1990). Use of pulmonary artery catheters in patients with acute myocardial infarction. Analysis of experience in 5,841 patients in the SPRINT Registry. SPRINT Study Group. *Chest* 98: 1331-35.

[20] Greenland P, Reicher-Reiss H, et al. (1991). In-hospital and one-year mortality in 1,524 women after myocardial infarction. Comparison with 4,315 men. *Circulation* 83: 484-91.

[21] Blumberg MS, Binns GS. (1994). Swan-Ganz catheter use and mortality of myocardial infarction patients. *Health Care Financ Rev* 15: 91-103.

[22] Cochrane Injuries Group Albumin Reviewers. (1998). Human albumin administration in critically ill patients: systematic review of randomised controlled trials. *BMJ* 317: 235-40.

[23] Offringa M. (1998). Excess mortality after human albumin administration in critically ill patients. Clinical and pathophysiological evidence suggests albumin is harmful. *BMJ* 317: 223-24.

[24] Offringa M (1998). Consider validity, clinical relevance, and applicability of albumin for critically ill patients. *BMJ* 317: 343.

[25] Heyland DK, MacDonald S, et al. (1998). Total parenteral nutrition in the critically ill patient: a meta-analysis. *JAMA* 280: 2013-19.

[26] Hebert PC, Wells G, et al. (1999). A multicenter, randomized, controlled clinical trial of transfusion requirements in critical care. Transfusion Requirements in Critical Care Investigators. Canadian Critical Care Trials Group. *N Engl J Med* 340: 409-17.

[27] Epstein AE, Hallstrom AP, et al. (1993). Mortality following ventricular arrhythmia suppression by encainide, flecainide, and moricizine after myocardial infarction. The original design concept of the Cardiac Arrhythmia Suppression Trial (CAST). *JAMA* 270: 2451-55.

[28] http://www.physweekly.com/archive/96/10_21_96/pc.html

Chapter Nine

The Dubious Merits of Screening for Cancer of the Breast and Prostate

Andrew Thompson, Norman J. Temple

In the previous chapter we questioned the value of statin drugs in dealing with coronary heart disease. This chapter will extend our skeptical reevaluation to screening and treatment procedures for breast and prostate cancer, two of the most prominent cancers in First World countries. Massive screening programs have been instituted for each, and these programs have been strongly promoted by health authorities, politicians, movie stars, and many other prominent persons. It is unorthodox, if not blasphemous, to take a contrary public stance. However, one important item has been overlooked in this juggernaut campaign. The research that has been done leaves serious question marks as to the value of screening for these cancers.

In theory, early detection of cancer permits early treatment which reduces the effect of the disease and increases the chances of a cure. Large amounts of time and money have been invested into this cancer-fighting strategy. But such investments – as in all areas of medicine – can easily lead to resistance to making an unbiased investigation. This is especially true if people make money and enhance their reputations by ignoring and downplaying evidence to the contrary and if it gives professionals and the public the illusion of success when there is none.

We start our critical analysis by examining the evidence for the value of mammography as a screening tool in the detection of breast cancer.

PART I: HAVE MAMMOGRAMS PROVEN THEIR VALUE?

Breast screening is an inherently inefficient health measure where it is not possible to strike a balance between economy, efficiency, and effectiveness. 'Finding it early' is detrimental to women's health and well

129

A. Thompson and N.J. Temple (eds.), Ethics, Medical Research, and Medicine, 129–145.
© 2001 *Kluwer Academic Publishers. Printed in the Netherlands.*

being.   Hazel Thornton, Consumers Advisory Group, Colchester, Great Britain[1]

Fear of cancer spurs much of today's medical expenses. Cancer is not just another disease, it is a dreaded disease, dreaded because it is associated with images of a foreign entity eating away at our body, an entity, which, if unchecked, will eventually devour enough tissue to strike a death blow at vital organs. And as the disease progresses so does the pain. Thus, it is no surprise that all a physician needs to do in order to persuade patients to agree to a diagnostic procedure or treatment is to raise the specter of cancer, letting fear do the rest. This certainly applies to breast cancer. Since it is common, any procedure routinely used to diagnose or treat it usurps a tremendous amount of resources, and, for that reason alone, should be assessed carefully.

Let us start by assuming that you are a woman and that you have heard on good authority that breast cancer is the second leading cause of death from cancer in women and that the incidence of it is increasing every year: an increase of 52 percent from cancer between 1950 and 1990 – this is after correcting for the increased number of older women.[2] As a result, one out of every eight women can be expected to develop breast cancer. But you have also heard that mammography can detect this cancer while it is still at an early stage, a stage when it can be successfully treated. Given this context, if your physician recommends you have yearly mammograms, you will most likely agree.

Now suppose, however, that your physician is a particularly honest, informed, and conscientious one who lets you know that the situation is not quite as presented and some facts ought to be added to make the picture complete. What might she tell you?

She might tell you that, on a yearly basis, the incidence of diagnosed breast cancer in the USA in 1990 was 109/100,000. A 52 percent increase from 1950 would mean that the incidence changed from 72 to 109 per 100,000 over a period of 40 years, or more simply stated, from almost one per 1000 to very slightly more than one per 1000.[2] Most would agree that this does not sound nearly as dramatic. (This does not mean breast cancer is not to be taken seriously, only that one has to beware of how statistics can be used to promote a "need to act now" campaign rather than to take the time to investigate the possible remedies in a thorough, careful manner.)

She further points out that much, and perhaps all, of this increase in incidence could be attributed to changes in screening and diagnosis. Mammography find suspicious shadows that might not otherwise be found, and diagnostic practices have changed in that small, local tumors, that are not clearly malignant and may never constitute a real problem, are now diagnosed as such and removed.[3,4,5,6]

Let's say you are under 50 years old. The physician decides to tell you that several studies on the efficacy of mammography have not found them to be of any use to your age group.[7,8,9] The breasts or tumors of that age group are different to those of older women, leading to inaccurate interpretation of the mammograms. And because of this there are a lot more "false positives" -- suspicious shadows that are investigated to see if they are malignant tumors and found not to be. In fact, for women in the 40 to 50 age group there are 2.5 times as many biopsies and three times as many diagnostic procedures to clear up suspicious findings as for older women. For every thousand women aged between 40 and 50 who have annual mammograms, it is estimated that a further diagnostic procedure will be required for 700 of them in a decade with the end result that 15 tumors will be found, but seven will remain undetected.[10]

Given all this information you may very well wonder at the wisdom of the recommendation by the American Cancer Society that women have regular mammograms beginning at age 40.[9]

Clearly, this is not the typical doctor-patient exchange over the value of mammography. Otherwise, 32 percent of American women in their 40s would not have had a mammogram in 1992.[7]

Now let's suppose you are 50 and you go back to your doctor. You have read that both the American Cancer Society and the National Cancer Institute recommend women of your age have regular screening that includes both clinical breast examinations and mammograms and you are wondering if you should start this regime. What additional facts might your unusually conscientious and informed doctor impart to you?

She might start by admitting that the whole basis for these recommendations is rather shaky. The only real proof of the value of breast screening would be long-term studies showing a significant reduction in risk of death from breast cancer when women are given mammography. But studies that have investigated mammography for the early detection of cancer are split between those that show a benefit and those that show none.[11] She also points out that some of the studies, including the widely publicized "positive" ones, may have had serious flaws in their design and execution, and that, as a result, the interpretation of the results was controversial.[12] Most importantly, the two studies judged to most credible in terms of their design and the ages of the participants found no effect of screening with mammography on breast cancer mortality.[13] In fact, one of these studies recently confirmed its earlier results based on more years of follow up.[14] This long-term study was carried out on almost 40,000 Canadian women aged 50 to 59 at the time of entry into the study. It found that adding annual mammography screening to annual, thorough, clinical breast examination does not lower breast cancer mortality.

Your doctor also warns you that the odds of having a false positive result from a mammogram are rather high. This results in having further diagnostic procedures such as additional mammograms or biopsies. A recent review, for example, found that there were 11 false positives for every finding that actually identified a tumor. Not surprisingly, women who undergo such procedures as a result of a false alarm often report anxiety about breast cancer, some 29 percent of them as much as 18 months later.[15]

Clearly, early screening is of no value unless there is effective treatment. But, the studies showing successful treatment of breast cancer, however detected, are themselves suspect. Lumpectomy, lumpectomy plus irradiation, and mastectomy all report the same level of survival rates, yet report different rates of reemergence of cancer: 30 percent for lumpectomy; 10 percent for lumpectomy plus irradiation; and zero percent for mastectomy.[11] These results are contradictory unless one assumes that the reemergence of cancer makes no difference to length of survival.

Even though the information your physician has given you flies in the face of the generally accepted "truth," you realize that she has nothing to gain by misleading you. You therefore decide to forego having any mammograms and rely instead on annual, thorough, clinical breast examinations.

Being a rather conscientious and inquisitive person, you wonder how much your physician has saved in expenses for your health insurance policy and how much this might be if extended over the general population of women. You are unable to get all the data but you do get some. You find out that the average mammogram costs $100 in the USA, and if you add in the average number of follow-up tests and biopsies of suspicious findings, the price becomes $128. This does not include office visits.[16] There are about 47 million women in the USA who some medical circles argue should have annual mammograms. That translates to over six billion dollars a year, or more than the total American expenditure for international development and humanitarian assistance.[17] You are astonished by this information and wonder how a medical procedure of such dubious value can be justified in view of other, clearly justifiable needs.

One way of looking at this expense is to compare the cost per life-year added by mammograms, with that of simply having clinical breast examinations. For this analysis we will make the dubious assumption that screening does indeed reduce the risk of death from breast cancer. Most cost-effectiveness studies concern themselves with the combined value of clinical breast examinations and mammograms but one expert separated out these two types of screening. According to one study, if the projections are based on a large, supportive, randomly controlled trial, it would cost from $84,000 to $134,081 per life-year gained (in 1985 dollars) to add mammograms to clinical breast examinations. A later, supportive, but uncontrolled study gives much lower figures, from $21,700 to $29,400.[18] Putting these figures in terms of quality life years and updating to year 2000 dollars would increase the costs considerably.

Another study lumps the clinical and the X-ray examinations together, as is customary. It also incorporated recent data indicating some benefits in terms of rate of survival from breast cancer for women aged 40 to 49. Nevertheless, it found the costs to be extremely high for this age group. The authors state: "To prevent one death among women aged 40 to 49 years of age, clinicians would have to routinely screen 2500 women."[19] The cost: $105,000 to $161,400 per added year of life. Annual screening of women aged 50 to 69 would cost a "modest" $45,000 per added year of life. A study on women aged 70 to 79 estimates that the cost is $117,700 per life-year gained.[20]

If these cost-analyses had been based on the two unbiased studies referred to earlier[13,14,21] that showed no advantage for mammography, then there would have been no point to doing a cost-analysis, since it would yield zero cost-effectiveness.

In any case, no matter what studies one uses, or how the cost-effectiveness is calculated, the costs for any age group of women would be much higher than the Proposed Standard of $25,000 (in year 2000 dollars) per quality life-year gained.

A last-ditch argument is that past, negative findings were not based on the latest, improved screening technology, and the new technology is sure to provide better, more positive results.[22] Following this logic to its conclusion, however, would result in never giving up on a technology, however valueless. Even if the new technology doesn't show any advantage in a clinical trial, or adds even more false positives, it can always be claimed that the next generation of high-tech screening devices (no doubt, already underway) will surely do better, ad infinitum.

The same faulty logic can be used to justify any similar questionable practice in medicine. The result would be that costs would continue to expand and soar with every new technology, regardless of its efficacy. The only way to stop this unaffordable and unethical process is to require that procedures and products are not marketed unless they are of proven value.

Currently, any efforts in this direction in the USA have been overridden by an aggressive campaign to persuade every woman over 40 to have an annual mammogram. This campaign has the support, even leadership, of nationally prominent people, and public pundits pass it on uncritically. The National Cancer Institute initially resisted the pressure to change its opinion that mammograms do not add anything before the age of 50, and, indeed, its advisory board recently recommended continuing this stance after again reviewing the available evidence. However, it was then faced with a strong protest led by some of the scientists who had submitted evidence and opinions, by breast cancer screening advocates, by members of Congress, and by the White House. The Senate passed a resolution supporting mammography in women aged 40 to 49 and the chair of the committee that funds NCI suggested it change its guidelines.[23]

This militancy is not limited to the USA, as evidenced by the experience of the Alusborg County Council in Sweden which, in the interest of cost saving, had decided to discontinue a breast-screening program for women aged 40 to 74. They intended to use these savings to pay for improved care for patients already suffering from cancer. The political opposition objected, and, with the help of doctors and various segments of the public, they forced a reversal of the decision. One 62-year old Member of Parliament even posed topless to illustrate an article opposing the relocation of funds.[24,25] However, at least for a moment, the wall was cracked.

Autologous Bone Marrow Transplantation

One treatment, originally intended only for women in the last stages of breast cancer, but then increasingly extended to others in response to public, professional, and political pressure, is Autologous Bone Marrow Transplantation (ABMT). This form of transplantation enables the body to absorb more chemotherapy without succumbing to its toxic effects. It was theorized that this would lead to more complete eradication of the malignant cells and, as reported in the early part of chapter four on publication biases, the initial Phase II trials did indicate this might be true. The resulting publicity led to the treatment being demanded by physicians and patients before the more reliable Phase III trials could be completed, and even interfered with their getting enough volunteers for these trials. Also, insurance companies were sued, some successfully, when they did not offer this unproven, very expensive ($49,000--$385,000) procedure.[26,27]

In preventive self-defense, Oregon Blue Cross Blue Shield instituted a procedure that embodies the ethical principle of informed consent from patients. It created a position of "Transplant Coordinator." An experienced nurse was appointed "whose job was to work directly with patients and families, transplant programs, employers, and the Oregon Blue Cross Blue Shield benefit systems to create mutually satisfactory individualized treatment plans. . . . [It] is an unusually open and accountable process of deliberation and reason-giving and an especially strong emphasis on supporting scientific treatment evaluation."[28] Patients are given articles to read concerning the treatment, and providers are challenged to make a scientific case for requests to pay for unproven procedures. If there are appropriate ongoing clinical trials on the procedure, patients are also given the option of becoming participants in them. If they agree, the plan will pay the costs. In randomized trials this would mean that they would have to risk being assigned to the group that receives conventional treatment or, in some cases, depending on the procedure, no treatment. According to the coordinator, as of June 1996, no patients had sued and many had decided that they didn't really want the unproven treatments that they had previously requested.

Since then, some of these trials have been completed, and, the results have been primarily negative. There has been sufficient publication of these results that the demand for ABMT has slackened considerably, at least according to the data gathered by a major insurer. It had an increase in the number of subscribers requesting ABMT from 64 to 83 per year between 1996 and 1998. But in 1999, after the publication of several studies showing no advantage for this treatment, only 42 subscribers requested the procedure, despite an increase in overall membership of 200,000.[29] If the Proposed Standards for research and publication had been followed, this information would have been available sooner and the misleading information would not have been "leaked" with all of the consequent costs to the public, both fiscal and in the subjecting of misinformed patients to this experimental and very painful treatment.

PART II: SCREENING FOR AND AGGRESSIVE TREATMENT OF PROSTATE CANCER

Routine screening for any condition is unwarranted without evidence that the test accurately detects early disease, that early detection improves outcomes, and that benefits outweigh harms. Unfortunately, such evidence is lacking for prostate cancer. Steven H. Woolf, associate clinical professor, Medical College of Virginia.[30]

The diagnosis and subsequent treatment of prostate cancer is not a proud chapter in the modern history of American medicine. However, it represents, better than other treatment approaches of which we are aware, what can and does go wrong when cancer phobia dominates the scene. For that reason we will explore the subject in some detail. As we shall see, the available evidence on diagnosis and treatment of prostate cancer does not support either set of procedures.

Let us start with how the statistics are presented. There are a great many articles on cancer of the prostate, many of which provide statistics on its incidence rate (the proportion of men affected) and on its mortality rate (the proportion of men dying from it). Based on these statistics, it is argued that prostate cancer is the most common type of cancer in men (the fact that skin cancer is more common is usually ignored, presumably because it is seldom fatal). However, with few exceptions, it is not the least bit clear what the evidence for this claim consists of. In one article it turned out that the evidence could include microscopic tumors discovered by autopsies, i.e., tumors that are so small and may be so slow growing that they may well not be the least bit dangerous within the subject's lifetime (Alexander). What proportion of the evidence is of this microscopic dimension is not clearly stated, only that over one third of men over 50 have at least microscopic evidence of prostate cancer.[31]

Presentation of the mortality rate is also variable and confusing. From our sampling of articles, the more frightening ones are the ones presented by the medical profession. To the degree that there is a consensus it is that most men, at least 70 percent of those who actually have cancer of the prostate gland (and not just microscopic evidence of it), will die with the disease and not from it. It is also clear that prostate cancer is strongly associated with age: the chance of getting it varies from less than one percent for men below age 50, to 50 percent for those above age 80.[32,33] Still that can be a frightening prospect for those who fear they may be stricken with the disease and they may very well want to improve their odds.

An apparently logical way to do so is to take the advice of the American Cancer Society and go to a physician for an annual checkup to detect early-stage prostate cancer, cancer when it is supposedly curable.[34] As we shall see, being "logical" in this case is to precipitate a potentially very expensive round of diagnostic testing leading to ineffective treatment.

Basically, there are two initial diagnostic tests. The first is the digital rectal examination (DRE) in which the physician inserts a gloved finger into the rectum and probes the prostate gland to determine if there are any suspicious lumps or other irregularities. A blood test may also be administered to measure the prostate-specific antigen level (PSA), especially if the DRE detects anything suspicious to the physician. If the level is above 4.0, it could indicate the presence of cancer; if above 10.0, it is "highly indicative" of the presence of cancer. If either test prompts concern on the part of the physician, further testing is likely.

One of the most likely next steps is to do an ultrasound-guided needle biopsy of several sections of the prostate, which material is then analyzed microscopically to determine the presence of cancer. If the results are positive, other tests are likely to be called for to further confirm the diagnosis and to determine the size, spread, and nature of any tumors. These include urinalysis, an extensive battery of additional blood tests, transrectal ultrasonography (TRUS), X-rays of the abdomen, and chest, intravenous pyelogram of the urinary system, and either a CAT or an MRI scan of the abdomen and pelvis. The TRUS, CAT, and MRI are especially expensive procedures.

One problem is that the DRE and the PSA tests, singly and together, are very inaccurate indicators of cancer. Individually, they provide considerable amount of false positives (indicating cancer when there is none) and false negatives (not detecting cancer that is present). Together, they don't do much better, with their overall diagnostic accuracy estimated by studies to be around 40 percent.[35,36] Knowing this, a lot of needle biopsies and other tests are apt to be ordered despite the likelihood that one is dealing with a false positive on one or both tests.

Unfortunately, needle biopsies have side effects which are apt to compound the diagnostic picture rather than resolve it. Since they are done through the rectum they can introduce bacteria from there into the prostate. Knowing this, antibiotics are typically also administered, but since the prostate is a poor medium for antibiotics, bacteria may survive and lead to a persistent, low-grade infection. This will raise the PSA level which, in turn, may be interpreted as further evidence of cancer, leading to more needle biopsies and still more infection, and so on. One way to check on this is to do a TRUS, which, however, has its own difficulties of interpretation. One study showed that only 70 percent of cancers were found when both it and biopsies were used, and it also produces false positives, thus leading to the need for still other tests even though no cancer is really present.[37] As with breast cancer, these false positives must create a huge burden of stress for those on the receiving end.

Now, suppose that enough of this battery of tests concurs and it is decided that you have prostate cancer. What happens next? If it has also been determined that your cancer is spread outside of the prostate and its immediate surrounding tissue, than you will be treated palliatively -- that is, various procedures, most notably hormonal therapy, will be introduced to reduce the size of the tumor and to relieve any distress you have.

If, however, you are one of the those whose cancer seems confined to the prostate gland, you are eligible for "aggressive" treatment designed to completely excise or kill the malignant tissue. In the USA radical prostatectomy, or surgical removal of the prostate gland, is the preferred option, possibly because it is urologists who typically first detect the cancer and then do the surgery. In the first part of the operation the lymph nodes are usually sampled to determine if the cancer has spread to them, and, if so, then the operation is canceled as being futile.

The operation requires a hospital stay of six days on average (some say more) and about 98 percent survive it (Alexander). If all goes well, one will be on a catheter for ten days which is connected to either a 700 mL "traveling bag" or to a 2000 mL stationary one. One then progresses to diapers, then shields. In six weeks most men are able to resume normal activity, albeit up to 50 percent may have intermittent loss of urine, and three to ten percent remain completely incontinent. Impotence characterizes most men who have this operation after the age of 70, but not the majority of younger men. However, at least a partial reduction of potency is expected in nearly all patients.[31,34,38]

One study shows that if you go to a radiation oncologist first, then radiation therapy is likely to be the procedure chosen (Alexander). The most common form of radiation therapy, and the one researched the most, is that of flooding the entire cancerous area with radiation ("external beam radiation"). It does not always kill all the cancerous cells but it could take 10 to 15 years for the tumor to return.

This therapy lasts for about six weeks and has numerous possible side effects including moderate to considerable fatigue, possible severe rectal pains with diarrhea and spasms, frequent urination accompanied with pain (a potentially permanent condition), and a two to three percent risk of damaging the bowel, bladder, or other organs. It also results in incontinence and impotence about as frequently as surgery.[32,34]

The newer form of radiation therapy (brachytherapy or interstitial radiation) requires insertion of radiation-emitting seeds or ribbons into the prostate, usually with the guidance of ultrasound. Strong beams of radiation are focused only on these areas, thus causing less general damage and less duration of radiation. But with this method there is less chance that all the cancerous spots will be located and reduced; thus broader beam radiation is often favored. Brachytherapy is also not without hazard and may cause erosion into the rectum and consequent partial interchange of urine and stool between the bladder and the rectum.[32] The most common side effects (10 percent each) are diarrhea and cystitis (inflammation of the bladder, usually accompanied by the desire to urinate frequently and a burning feeling when one does so). Less common, but significant, are inflammation of the rectum, rectal bleeding, blood in the urine, impotence, and incontinence.[34]

The radical treatments and the diagnostic tests which precede them are, needless to say, highly expensive. The American Cancer Society recommends annual screening of all white men over 50 and all black men over 40. Just a one-time screening of all men over 50 would cost $7 to $28 billion, plus $3 billion for each subsequent year.[30] Since 1994 there have been over 100,000 radical prostatectomies performed per year in the USA, at a cost of about $25,000 per operation, or over $2.5 billion per year. We do not have comparable figures for radiation therapy that is intended to eliminate the cancer, but it could add at least $1 billion.[39,40] By comparison, the cost to eliminate Russia's stockpile of chemical weapons, the world's largest, is $5.5 billion – something Russia says it is willing to do it if it could afford it.[41] The entire US estimated federal outlay for 1999 for natural resources and the environment is less than $24 billion and that for community and regional development, including disaster relief and insurance, is $11 billion.[42]

The justification for all this tremendous outpouring of money, that could be used in uncounted other, clearly justifiable ways, is simple -- it saves men from dying of prostate cancer. But does it really, and even if it does extend the lives of some men, is it worth it in terms of the quality of their extended life? These questions have been called into play by several studies, the most important of which are the following two: The Swedish Study and the Veteran's Administration Study.[34,35,43,44]

In the Swedish Study 223 patients with early-stage prostate cancer, whose average age was 72, were left untreated until such time as the cancer spread was evident. They then received hormone treatment to relieve the symptoms. Of those who had died after ten years,19 percent had died of prostate cancer and the rest of other causes. These mortality rates were not significantly different from that of another group of 77 patients who were initially treated with local irradiation, estrogen, estramustine, removal of one or both testes, or a combination of these treatments.

The Swedish study has been attacked as being unrepresentative in that its subjects were older and had mostly low-grade cancers. This and other criticisms were not supported by a pooled analysis of six studies whose patients had a much younger average age and higher-grade cancers.[45]

In the Veteran's Administration Study 111 patients with operable prostate cancer were divided into two groups. One group was placed on placebo and the other had surgery. Fifteen years later there was no difference in the mortality rate of the two groups due to cancer. Also, there was no difference between the mortality rate of these patients and that of the general male population.[46] Thus, neither having prostate cancer nor having surgery for it affected life expectancy. The study has been criticized as being too small but the results are not indicative that having more participants would have made a difference. Also, it is the only randomized, controlled study making this comparison.

The results of the Veterans and the Swedish studies are also consistent with the fact that the mortality rate due to prostate cancer has not changed in recent years despite the increased detection of early-stage cancer and the boom in aggressive treatment of this kind of cancer.[35] For instance, the reported incidence rate suddenly doubled between 1986 and 1991. This clearly reflects mass screening. Yet there was no particular favorable trend in mortality rate for this disease in the years up to 1996.[47]

There are other studies, but not full-scale clinical trials. An article and an editorial in the *Journal of the American Medical Association* pointed out that even if one assumed the studies showing the most favorable results from aggressive treatment were credible, it is questionable that the quality of life would be better for those undergoing surgery or radiation than for those who forego such treatment.[48,49] Also, the length of life would be at most one year more on average, but then only for the younger men. If the studies showing negative results were used to make these projections instead, even this dubious advantage of aggressive treatment would disappear. It is noteworthy that Great Britain's national health system does not pay for screening for prostate cancer, in view of the lack of evidence that such screening accurately detects early disease or that early detection improves outcomes.[30,50]

Because of these and other similar findings the National Cancer Institute decided that a definitive study needs to be conducted to determine the value, if any, of screening for prostate cancer. It recently instigated a 16-year, multicenter, controlled study to this effect.[34] However, the researchers have been unable to recruit enough participants in the study, with the result that the whole study is in jeopardy.[51] The problem seems to be that when prospective volunteers are told they could be randomly assigned to the "watchful waiting" group rather than to the aggressive treatment one, they are not willing to take the risk since they believe aggressive treatment to be effective. Fortunately, there is one other major randomized study underway in Scandinavia.[52]

Some recent articles in medical journals have underscored the need for this type of study. One can only hope the medical profession will begin to promote it or that the media will pick up on the issue and quit promoting aggressive treatment with illustrated articles about prominent men who had "successful" prostate cancer surgery or who are courageously fighting for their lives by undergoing it.[30,53,54]

CONCLUDING COMMENTS

We have looked at the standard screening programs for breast and prostate cancer, two of the most common forms of cancer in First World countries, in terms of both incidence and mortality. Neither had to undergo any rigorous test of its efficacy before becoming an established practice. Both cost many billions of dollars to implement, yet, at least in the United States, both are aggressively and enthusiastically promoted. And, in both cases, there is no good evidence that the treatments that they lead to are of any real value. The evidence that is sometimes offered is that five-year survival rates have improved for most, if not all, cancers. An article critiquing this practice[55] started with this example from a recent press release from the US Department of Health and Human Services:

> *The five-year survival rate for all cancers improved from 51 percent in the early 1980s to almost 60 percent in the early 1990s . . .since the 1971 National Cancer Act, much of the research into early cancer detection and treatment has paid off.*

The article went on to point out that survival rates may be extremely misleading for three reasons: lead-time bias caused by early detection, hence a longer period of time for the disease to develop before the five years are up; changed diagnostic procedures that diagnose more tumors as malignant or potentially so; and improvement in the treatment of the disease over the years.

What is lead-time bias? Here is an example, an extreme case based on an imaginary cancer. Previously, the cancer was not detected until after clinical symptoms appeared. The cancer is incurable and death always followed three years after clinical symptoms. However, screening has been introduced so that the cancer is now diagnosed three years before clinical symptoms appear. Alas, no new treatments are available. As a result of screening, the time gap between diagnosis and death lengthens from three years to six. Even more miraculously the five-year survival goes from zero to one hundred percent! Something of this has taken place with several types of cancer leading to a spurious increase in the five-year survival rate.

Incidence rates are also misleading because they also change according to changes in diagnostic procedures and policies. Thus, tumors which before would not have been found, or if found, would not have been judged malignant, may now be classified as malignant. When this is done, and yet the same number die from the cancer, then it appears as if treatment is more successful when it really is not.

The gold standard way of determining success in a treatment approach, including one involving early screening and treatment, is to examine trends in mortality rates. If improvements in five-year survival are real, then improved survival should be reflected in lowered mortality (but with little or no change in incidence). The above article, however, found little correlation between five-year survival rates and mortality rates for 20 solid tumors. This is consistent with there being little value to early screening and treatment, at least for most cancers.

By contrast, there was a strong correlation between five-year survival and incidence. This indicates that both have been artificially inflated by widespread over-diagnosis of cancer. In other words there is an epidemic of nonexistent cancer and each such case is counted in both the "survival" and "incidence" tallies.

Prostate cancer showed a slight increase in age-adjusted mortality and breast cancer showed a slight decrease. These modest changes could be the result of differences in treatment over the years, in the former case the increase in aggressive treatment, and in the latter, improvements in chemotherapy treatment; or it could be a true change in incidence.

The paper by Welch provides strong evidence, therefore, that the war against cancer is not being won. That claim is far from new. For instance, Bailar and Gornik[56] also made this claim, though using a different line of argument.

It is no secret that the best, most reliable way to determine success in medical treatment of life-shortening diseases is to calculate mortality rates in clinical trials, especially, as we have argued, overall mortality rates in long-term trials which compare the new, experimental procedures to recommended ones. Why hasn't this come to pass, other than in a delayed and infrequent manner? Why are biased statistics used instead, statistics that apparently show splendid progress where little or none exists? There are many reasons, two of the major ones being that money and careers are made by the promotion of these screening tests and the subsequent treatments.

The mind-sets of public officials and of physicians could also be important here. The public officials that have promoting screening so vigorously do not want to lose face by admitting they have been overeager to do something that looked promising instead of demanding proper evidence in advance. Thus they cover up their mistaken judgment by using misleading statistics and continue to support this continuing drain of resources. Physicians have also rushed to judgment. They want to provide hope to their cancer patients and have ignored evidence that contradicts what they do not want to hear. Some of this evidence, such as the long-term studies on treatment for prostate cancer, has been available for a long time, but has been largely ignored or downplayed by urologists and radiologists in the USA in particular. This is a field that warrants a lot of skepticism and much more promotion of guidelines for research and publication, such as we have proposed, if the public is truly to realize any benefit rather than a drain on resources.

After all the many, many success stories reported over the years in the war against cancer, we are entitled, perhaps, to ask one question: If things are so good, why are they so bad?

References

Part I: Breast Cancer:

[1] Thornton H (1998). Breast cancer screening. *Lancet* 351:145

[2] CDC (1994). Death from breast cancer -- United States, 1991. *JAMA* 271:1395.

[3] Hakama M, Kaija H, et al. (1995). Aggressiveness of screen-detected breast cancers. *Lancet* 314: 221-23.

[4] Nab HW, Wim CJ, et al. (1994). Changes in long term prognosis for breast cancer in a Dutch cancer registry. *BMJ* 309: 83-86.

[5] Thomas BA (1995). Population breast cancer screening: theory, practice, and service implications. *Lancet* 345: 205-07.

[6] Feuer EJ, Lap-Ming W (1992). How much of the recent rise in breast cancer incidence can be explained by increases in mammography utilization? *Am J Epidemiol* 136:1423-36.

[7] Kolata G (February 26, 1993). Do mammograms aid women in 40s? *New York Times*: 1A, 4A.

[8] Kerlikowske K (1997). Efficacy of screening mammography among women aged 40 to 49 years and 50 to 69 years: comparison of relative and absolute benefit. *J Natl Cancer Inst Monogr* No. 22: 79-86.

[9] Kattlove H, Alessandro L, et al. (1995). Benefits and costs of screening and treatment for early breast cancer. *JAMA* 273: 142-48.

[10] Davis DL (1994). Mammographic screening. *JAMA* 271: 152-53.

[11] Devitt JE (1994). Breast cancer: have we missed the forest because of the tree? *Lancet* 344: 734-35.

[12] Shapiro S (1992). Periodic breast cancer screening in seven foreign countries. *Cancer* 69 (*suppl 7*): 1919-24.

[13] Gotzsche PC, Olsen O (2000). Is screening for breast cancer with mammography justifiable? *Lancet* 355: 129-34.

[14] Miller AB, To T, et al. (2000). Canadian National Breast Screening Study-2: 13-Year Results of a Randomized Trial in Women Aged 50–59 Years. *J Natl Cancer Inst* 92: 1490-99.

[15] Elmore JG, Barton MB, et al. (1998). Ten-year risk of false positive screening mammograms and clinical breast examinations. *N Engl J Med* 338:1089-96.

[16] Mushlin AI, Fintor L (1992). Is screening for breast cancer cost-effective? *Cancer* 69 (*suppl 7*): 1957-62

[17] CQ Staff (February 7, 1998). How each agency and department would fare under Clinton budget. *CQ*: 297-314.

[18] Eddy, DM (1989). Screening for breast cancer. *Ann Intern Med* 111: 389-99.

[19] Salzmann P, Kerlikowske K (1997). Cost-effectiveness of extending mammography guidelines to include women 40 to 49 years of age. *Ann Intern Med* 127: 955-64.

[20] Kerlikowske K, Grady D, et al. (1995). Efficacy of screening mammography: a meta-analysis. *JAMA* 273: 149-154.

[21] Andersson I, Aspergren K, et al. (1988). Mammographic screening and mortality from breast cancer: the Malmo mammographic screening trial. *BMJ* 297: 943-58.

[22] Sickles E A, Kopans DB (1995). Mammographic screening for women aged 40 to 49 years: the primary care practitioner's dilemma. *Ann Intern Med* 122: 534-38.

[23] Woolf SH, Lawrence RS (1997). Lessons from the consensus panel on mammography screening. *JAMA* 278: 2105-08.

[24] Awuonda M (1996). Swedish county criticized for halting breast screening. *Lancet* 347: 608.

[25] Awuonda M (1996). Swedes in volte-face on breast screening. *Lancet* 347: 822.

[26] Triozi PL (1994). Autologous bone marrow and peripheral blood progenitor transplant for breast cancer. *Lancet* 344: 418-19.

[27] Peters WP, Rogers MC (1994). Variation in approval by insurance companies of coverage for autologous bone marrow transplantation for breast cancer. *N Engl J Med* 330: 473-77.

[28] Daniels N, Sabin JE (March-April, 1998). Last chance therapies and managed care. *Hastings Center Report*: 27-41.

[29] v. Amerongen D (2000). (Letter to the editor). Insurance payments for bone marrow transplantation in metastatic breast cancer. *N Engl J Med* 342: 1138-39.

Part II: Prostate Cancer:

[30] Woolf SH (1997). Should we screen for prostate cancer? *BMJ* 314: 989-90.

[31] Frydenberg M, Stricker PD, (1997). Prostate cancer diagnosis and management. *Lancet* 349: 1681-86.

[32] Zinner N R (1991). In: Dollinger M, Rosenbaum EH, Cable G, eds. *Everyone's guide to cancertherapy*. New York: Andrews and McNeil.

[33] Early prostate cancer best left alone -- treatment riskier than cancer. July 1993. *Health Facts*: 1,4.

[34] Alexander T (September 20, 1993). One man's tough choices on prostrate cancer. *Fortune*: 86-99.

[35] Cupp M R, Oesterling JE (1993). Prostate-specific antigen, digital rectal examination, and transrectal ultrasonography: their roles in diagnosing early prostate cancer. *Mayo Clinic Proc* 68: 297-306.

[36] Edelstein R A, Babayan RK (April 15, 1993). Managing prostate cancer, Part I: Localized Disease. *Hospital Practice*: 61-8, 70, 75-81.

[37] Brawer M K (1993). The diagnosis of prostatic carcinoma. *Cancer* 71: 899-905.

[38] National Cancer Institute (March 4, 1994). *PDQ state-of-the-art cancer treatment information: prostate cancer*.

[39] Mulley AG, Barry MJ (1998). Controversy in managing patients with prostate cancer. *BMJ* 316: 1919-20.

[40] Grady D (May 6,1999). New method gauges risk of prostate cancer relapse. *International Herald Tribune*.

[41] Hoffman D (September 27, 1998). Cold War's wastes lie buried in Russia. *Register-Guard*, Eugene, OR: 14A-15A.

[42] CQ Staff (February 7, 1998). How each agency and department would fare under Clinton budget. *CQ*: 297-314.

[43] Johansson J-E, Andersson S-O, et al. (1989). Natural history of localized prostatic cancer. *Lancet* 1: 799-803.

[44] Johansson J-E, Hohmberg L, et al. (1997). Fifteen year survival in prostate cancer: a prospective, population-based study in Sweden. *JAMA* 277: 467-71.

[45] Chodak GW (1994). The role of watchful waiting in the management of localized prostate cancer. *J Urology* 152: 1766-72.

[46] Graversen PH, Nielsen KT (1990). Radical prostatectomy versus expectant primary treatment in stages I and II. *Urology* 36: 493-98.

[47] Greenlee RT, Murray S, et al. (2000). Cancer Statistics. *Ca* 50: 7-33.

[48] Fleming C, Wasson JH, et al. (1993). A decision analysis of alternative treatment strategies for clinically localized prostate cancer. *JAMA* 269: 2650-58.

[49] Whitmore WF (1993). Management of clinically localized prostatic cancer: An unresolved problem. *JAMA* 269: 2676-77.

[50] Morris K (1997). UK experts advise against prostate cancer screening. *Lancet* 349: 477.

[51] Kolata G (February 13, 1997). Prostate study lacks volunteers. *International Herald Tribune*: 11.

[52] Dearnaly DP, Melia J (1997). Early prostate cancer — to treat or not? *Lancet* 349: 892-93.

[53] Collins MM, Barry MJ (1996). Controversies in prostate cancer screening. *JAMA* 276:1976-79.

[54] Raffle AE (1996). Trust me, I'm a scientist: Will urologists set a lead for geneticists to follow? *Lancet* 347: 883-84.

[55] Welch HG, Schwartz, LM, Woloshin S (2000). Are increasing 5-year survival rates evidence of success against cancer? *JAMA* 283: 2975-78.

[56] Bailar JC, Gornik HL (1997). Cancer undefeated. *N Engl J Med* 336: 1569-74.

Chapter Ten

The Genomics Revolution in Medicine: A Case of Extreme Information Overload

Andrew Thompson, Norman J. Temple

"The cure is just around the corner" mentality has been given a dynamic boost and new meaning by what might be called "the age of the genome." Any and every currently unconquered chronic condition and debilitating disease can conceivably be vanquished by the new technology -- even aging. Our daily informational diet is spiced with announcements, television programs, editorials, and magazine articles promoting new, possible cures and enhancements of the human condition. We are told that we are on the threshold of a marvelous new world where we will unlock the secrets of life and improve on it in almost every conceivable way, ranging from conquering disease to growing vitamin-rich, disease-resistant, fast-growing, new crops, to cleaning up our wastes by genetically-engineered bacteria. Exciting times indeed for scientists involved in this epic research and for those of us with great expectations.

In this chapter we explore selected aspects of how the genomics revolution is being applied to medicine. One aspect of this is using a detailed knowledge of a person's genes in order to predict diseases that they may be vulnerable to. However, the main focus of attention is on developing new therapies based on genomics. This medical strategy is often referred to as "gene therapy." It includes switching genes on or off, as appropriate, inserting new genes, and discovering the products of genes so that new drugs can be developed (for instance, by replacing a natural substance that a person may be failing to produce or by blocking the action of a substance that is being produced but is undesirable).

Before we make a detailed examination of gene therapy, we should step back and look at some broader principles. One of us (NT) has for a number of years argued that medical research can be divided into two types: complex and simple.[1,2,3] The words "complex" and "simple" refer to the degree of complexity in translating observations into practical knowledge that can be

147

A. Thompson and N.J. Temple (eds.), Ethics, Medical Research, and Medicine, 147–168.
© 2001 *Kluwer Academic Publishers. Printed in the Netherlands.*

applied to problems of human health. Complex research includes most studies on disease mechanisms. It most often leads not to light at the end of the tunnel but to more tunnels where the light should be. Simple research, by contrast, includes epidemiological studies, such as comparisons of disease incidence and lifestyle factors across populations, as well as human intervention trials. Simple research has given us the bulk of our practical knowledge. For instance, our understanding of the role of diet, exercise, and smoking in the cause and prevention of chronic diseases has come almost entirely from simple research. Yet, the lion's share of research dollars goes instead to studies of disease mechanisms.

By far the biggest area where complex research dominates is cancer. Research on this disease demonstrates how it is possible to spend over a billion dollars year after year and yet make trivial progress. Aspects of this were discussed in the previous chapter.

Gene therapy shows all the signs of repeating the mistakes of cancer research but on a grander scale. What we see is vast spending on complex research and regular announcements of "breakthroughs." However, based on the track record of complex research, we must be pessimistic over the likelihood that gene therapy will lead to real progress in finding cures for disease. Gene therapy seems well on its way to becoming the greatest sinkhole for research dollars.

This viewpoint is reinforced by a consideration of the relative importance of heredity as a cause of disease. Implicit in gene therapy is the assumption that disease is somehow caused by faulty genes, or at least that the genes are not behaving themselves. However, migration studies have convincingly shown that environmental factors dominate over genetic ones in the causation of chronic disease. For instance, large numbers of Japanese migrated from Japan to Hawaii and California early in the twentieth century. They adopted the diet and lifestyle of their new home. Over time, their disease pattern shifted from a Japanese one to an American one: there was a dramatic increase in such diseases as cancer of the colon and breast, while stomach cancer, previously very common, declined sharply. Since the 1950s Japan itself has adopted a more American lifestyle and this has led to the same trends in disease rates as seen in Japanese migrants to the USA.

While genetic factors undoubtedly play a role in disease causation, their importance has been much exaggerated. Much of the problem originates in interpretation of twin studies. For instance, numerous studies have shown that identical twins who grow up apart much resemble each other in such areas as weight. From this it is deduced that genes plays a much stronger role in causing obesity and numerous other conditions than does lifestyle. But this logic has a flaw. It ignores the fact that it is our environment that causes disease and we all live in more or less the same environment. Take obesity. We are all surrounded by fattening foods and few adults are forced to exercise. Who gets obesity is then determined by our genes. The same goes for heart disease and other diseases that run in families. If we take away the pathogenic environment, no one will get these diseases, regardless of their genes. We can illustrate this with the following example. A man visits his physician who tells him bluntly that he is fat. "But it's my genes, doctor. Being fat runs in my family." The physician replies: "Yes, you're fat, your wife is fat, and your kids are fat. Even your dog is fat. Obesity runs in your family!"

A recent study of twins, probably the best ever done, provides the corrective influence.[4] The investigators studied the role of heredity in cancer in 28 anatomical sites for almost 45,000 twins listed in the Swedish, Danish, and Finnish twin registries. Statistically significant effects of heritable factors were found only for three cancers: prostate, colorectal, and breast. The effects were higher, of course, for identical twins. The proportion of all men with prostate cancer whose twin also had prostate cancer was 21 percent for identical twins and only 6 percent for fraternal twins. The corresponding figures for women with breast cancer were 14 percent and nine percent; for men with colorectal cancer, it was nine percent and eight percent; and for women with colorectal cancer it was 16 percent and six percent. In short, in each case the role of environmental factors was much greater than that of heredity, even for the few "heritable cancers."

The editorial writer who commented on this article added another little tidbit: "A woman's average annual risk of a contralateral breast cancer after the diagnosis of a first primary breast cancer is about 0.8 percent — and this risk is for a person with, obviously, not only the identical genome, but also the identical complex of exposures."[5] Now some other diseases and conditions show a stronger hereditary component, but, such definitive twin studies have not been done to tell us how much.

In the great majority of cases, therefore, the dominant cause of disease lies in our environment and lifestyle, not in our genes. Since the 1970s great progress has been made in our understanding of the factors that cause or prevent disease, especially chronic diseases. As a result we are in a position now to prevent a large fraction of these chronic diseases. Less frequently, this knowledge has also led to exciting progress in finding new and effective therapies as is the case with obesity, heart disease, and hypertension. The reason for this rapid progress in finding ways to prevent disease – as was discussed above – is that it is based on simple research, especially epidemiology.

Based on this reasoning – and before we even begin a detailed exploration of gene therapy – we must express the view that in terms of getting the biggest bang for the research buck, simple research into ways to prevent and treat disease holds out far, far greater promise than does gene therapy research.

GENES AND GENE THERAPY

Before we succumb to the avalanche of promises it may be best to give them a context, one that grounds us in reality rather than being kept in a passive role due to awe of the science involved, awe based partly on our inability to comprehend much of what is claimed, only the claims themselves. Let us start with what most of us have been told several times, probably only to forget much of it. The nucleus of every cell contains 23 pairs of chromosomes, each of which contains genetic material in the form of two intertwining strands of DNA (deoxyribonucleuic acid), a "double helix." Each strand consists of a long series of "bases" called "A" (adenine), "C" (cytosine), "G" (guanine), and "T" (thymine). If uncoiled, a strand would be about six feet long. G on one chain always faces a C on the other, and A faces T, and these are referred to as "base pairs." Thus, all that is needed to know what is in the complimentary strand is to know the sequence in one of them. The strands are laid on a molecular scaffolding. Sequences of bases "code" for amino acids which are then assembled into proteins. Every three bases corresponds to one amino acid. Thus, when a gene is "switched on," the DNA is "read" and this acts as a blueprint for the building of a protein. The proteins, in turn, perform the process that carries out the gene's function. In the theatre of the cell, DNA is the script and proteins are the actors.

This all sounds fairly straightforward and represents an impressive array of knowledge, albeit complex. Some of the words such as "code," "switch on," and "read" are disturbing because their actual content is murky, but one presumes that the scientists involved understand the processes that these words represent. As you will soon see, this is not really the case. For one thing, only about three percent of the sequences "represent" the instructions for all the proteins made in the body. The remainder are in the relatively vast regions that separate the known genes, and their function is unknown. John Sulston[6], director of the United Kindgom's Sanger Centre in Cambridge, one of the centers involved in mapping the human genome, said: "We don't know what's junk and what isn't. We have no way of passing DNA through a machine that tells us what is junk." This unknown portion and the unknown aspects of the functioning of our genome has occupied the thinking of Christoph Rehmann-Sutter, a molecular biologist who went on to study philosophy and sociology and then founded the Institute for History and Ethics of Medicine at the University of Basel in Switzerland.[7] Let us see what he has to say.

Rehmann-Sutter starts his analysis by disabusing us of the notion that all is fixed, stable, and predictable in the human genome. Rather than in a tightly bound structure, the bases that constitute the sequences are typically scattered on the DNA molecular structure. In between these bases are other molecules that don't seem to belong and whose function is unknown. Identifying the gene sequences was thus an incredible task in itself, but only the beginning of even more incredible tasks. One has to identify the protein that goes with a gene since the protein does the work of the gene. But when and where this protein is built, how it is integrated with other molecules, and how it is synthesized and regulated by local constellations is not within our knowledge bank, and finding such things out cannot be done automatically by computers, such as sequencing is. Worse yet, the sequences themselves are sometimes changed when translated by the proteins. These changes are due to various environmental factors such as other molecules, concentrations of waste material, or the molecular scaffolding. When and how the gene switches on its protein depends on still other unknown factors. In short, the organism is not controlled by its DNA, nor does the organism control its DNA. Rather, there is an ongoing interaction, an interaction which varies according to the developmental stage of all its components, including the death and birth of new cells.

It is therefore clear - and this is about the only thing that is clear - that we have only made the down payment on the mortgage which, when paid off, will supposedly allow us to comprehend the mystery of life itself. Getting this far was not easy. The discovery of the double helix structure of DNA was made in 1953. Progress therefore occurs over decades. In recent years it took 1100 scientists in four large sequencing laboratories in the USA, plus others in five other countries in this $250 million the publicly-funded project just to "map" the base pairs.[8] The project also attracted a fortune in private venture capital, including a rival, privately-funded genome project using a different method which provides somewhat different data – at a price. As of 1998, there were 170 companies in the USA alone who were directly involved in gene therapy research and development, most financed by risk capital, with a total investment of between $800 and $900 million.[9] This far exceeds the public sector's contribution of about $200 million a year. In fact, private companies are sponsoring most of the clinical trials and "many academic centers have created gene-therapy programs and joined the jockeying for a piece of the action."[10]

We could easily expend many, many times that in terms of use of scientists, resources, and money in the effort to find out more. Is it worth the effort? Let us look at some of the promises that are made in this field of medicine and the results that have been realized so far to find answers to this question.

DIAGNOSIS BY DNA COMPUTER CHIPS

Advances in gene research promise — at least in theory — to provide people with accurate knowledge of all the diseases to which they may be subject because of their genes. With this knowledge people should be able to take measures so as to prevent the development of these crippling conditions. If prevention fails, then precisely-targeted treatments will be available. This "Brave New World" is an irresistible promise, typically made in an authoritative manner. But how realistic are these claims?

One of the questions that should be asked is: How much would a complete diagnosis cost? It is not a popular question and the data for answering it are sparse. It is clear that a complete genetic diagnosis is not likely to be widely affordable. For example, one company sells a set of computer chips (files) for $10,000 which represents about 7000 genes. When we consider that there are somewhere between 40,000 and 100,000 genes in the human genome, it is obvious that far more computer chips will be needed to do anything like a complete genetic diagnosis of an individual.[11]

Another problem is the accuracy of any such diagnosis. For example, applying one of the chips to bone marrow samples resulted in 29 out of 34 correct distinctions between two different types of leukemia. This may sound good but a 15 percent error rate is not exactly what one would expect from such a sophisticated and expensive technology and can lead to a lot of grief.[11] There are also some "technical problems." Oncormed, a genetic testing company, recently learned that one of its tests had rather adverse effects. A woman tested for breast cancer genes was told that she had inherited a mutation that put her at increased risk of breast and ovarian cancer. Consequently, she had her ovaries removed. A second test, eight months later, found no such mutation.[12] Even when the mutated gene is known (the disease-causing gene), routine genetic testing may fail to identify mutations in 25 to 75 percent or more of cases.[13] In other words, the tested person has little assurance that they don't have the gene in question. An example is provided by German Cancer Help. This organization concluded that given the rarity of BRCA 1 and BRCA 2, the two genes associated with breast cancer, it is unlikely that general population screening of women for these genes would be efficient. Therefore, it commissioned a study to assess the predictability of genetic testing on women who had at least three relatives who had died of breast cancer. The testing was not useful even for this select group since it did not show a specially high risk of breast cancer for them. This, despite the fact that epidemiological studies predict that one out of every two of them will get breast cancer. Nevertheless, commercial firms market the test for breast cancer for $2,000.[14] None of this is very reassuring about the value of such testing or of the ethics of those who market it. Unless there is some sort of stringent quality control is put in place and a great deal more accuracy obtained, such testing is arguably worse than useless.

But even if such accuracy was achieved, what good would it do you to have your own personal DNA test for a group of diseases? The answer is not obvious because the knowledge that is gained is neither simple nor immediately useful. In fact, it is likely to be more confusing and worrisome than helpful. As was stressed earlier, the role of genes in disease has probably been much exaggerated. It is estimated that there are around 3,000 single gene or "gene-specific" diseases. Having a gene that creates a disposition to a particular disease is a long way from saying that you will actually suffer from it. For a start, you can have the gene for a disease but it may never "express" itself during your lifetime, even if it is the sole gene that induces the disease. Even with single-gene defects its contribution to the occurrence of disease may be quite minor. But contrary to media-promoted impressions, single-gene defects, are, relatively speaking, not very common. Knowing this, we should be less impressed with the daily announcements of the discovery of a gene that is "responsible" for a given disease or condition. In reality, most genetic defects are thought to be of multigenetic origin. Just to identify all the genes involved in such multigenetic defects and determine their interaction may well be an impossible task[15,16] For most diseases or conditions, there are likely to be several, perhaps many, genes that contribute to it. How many of the genes associated with, for example, prostate cancer are causally related remains to be seen, but even if it is only a tiny number, say half a dozen, that still poses tremendous problems of interpretation when we deal with individual men. Most likely, each gene's contribution is very minor. For example, 50 genes were used in the DNA chip to identify, inaccurately, which of two types of leukemia the individuals had.

Let us now suppose that all this information has been fully deciphered. Each individual will most likely be found to have several, perhaps hundreds, of "predispositional genes," genes that create a partial disposition for having a particular disease. How does one convey such information in a useful and accurate fashion to individuals that are "fortunate" enough to have a fairly complete DNA diagnostic work-up? In actuality, the total information made available is both too imprecise and too much to be conveyed in either an accurate or an understandable manner. Over and over again, the physician or genetic counselor, assuming he or she was sufficiently honest and modest, would have to say: "There is a 10 to 90 percent chance that you will come down with this disease during your lifetime. How great the percentage is depends on a number of factors that we don't know how to weigh and may not be under your control in any case, and many of which are unknown to us." Even for one of the few "sure to be expressed genes," such as the one for Huntington's disease, they cannot predict with any precision when it is likely to emerge, how severe it will be, or its progress, and only 95 percent sure it will emerge before you die, even if you reach the age of 70.[8,17] The counseling situation, already difficult for the "simpler," strongly gene-influenced diseases, will become impossible with the addition of the plethora of other conditions that will have some genetic roots, most of which are multiple, but dominated by lifestyle factors.

For example, even now, counseling for just one genetic condition, hereditary non-polyposis colorectal cancer, poses problems. In order to see if it were possible to reduce the number of counseling sessions, a study was conducted which found that all that most subjects needed was one pretest session, a two-week reflection period, and a test-disclosure session, with more sessions available upon request. The pre- and post-test sessions were described as "absolutely necessary."[18] Two diseases may well require more than twice as much counseling because of questions about the possible interaction of the two diseases. Since everyone is bound to have multiple genetic predispositions, we can therefore predict that in any large sampling of genetically-linked diseases, the result is foredoomed: for most clients understanding their situation will be like trying to do a jumbo crossword puzzle in Russian.

One highly touted discovery was of finding genes associated with Alzheimer's disease. Yet a recent book points out that no predictive test for the typical late-onset (after age 65) form of Alzheimer's disease exists and the early-onset cases (before age 55) constitute only one to two per cent of the total afflicted.[19] Even then, the book is negative about the usefulness of genetic testing for this younger population, and for good reason. No genetic test will guarantee that the disease will strike: environmental factors as well as still unidentified genes are almost certainly involved.[20]

What is not typically pointed out is that there is no real value in genetic diagnosis unless it results in efficacious treatment. But what genetic diagnosis typically provides is a lot of information, some of it even patently false, as in the case of faulty diagnoses, and the rest of confusing complexity.[21] The diagnostic information will inevitably result in increased discrimination in obtaining employment and in procuring affordable health insurance for those whose genetic profile is not deemed to be optimal.[21,22]

GENETICALLY-ENGINEERED DRUGS

There is no end to claims about the value of genomic studies. They can aid in learning how diseases progress, and this in turn might enable scientists to find ways of interrupting the process at an earlier, more effective time. Genomic studies can also aid in the development of more precise diagnosis of diseases, as we have discussed with regard to DNA chips. This could lead to the design of new chemicals that would potentially modify a wide variety of biological functions. For example, substances could be designed that switch off the "bad" genes or switch on the "good" ones.[23] What seldom accompanies these promissory notes is an honest and more than cursory assessment of the overwhelming difficulties that would have to be overcome to make good on them.

It is theoretically possible to make individual-specific diagnoses. The form of the disease that the individual has could be identified, and the appropriate drug, especially engineered for that form of the disease, could then be given.[11] However, things are not as simple as they sound. The unit of measurement that is crucial to the success of a particular treatment is smaller than a gene. It often consists of the placement of a single "letter" (A, T, C, or G) in a single sequence in a person's genome. If you have a T where your neighbor has a C, then that might cause a difference in a reaction to a drug.[8] These letters are also called single-nucleotide polymorphisms (SNPs). The total number of SNPs in the human genome is estimated at one million. Just to determine which ones will alter the gene's protein product or its expression is a daunting task. For one reason, most of these difference-causing SNPs will be found in less than a few percent of the human population. Detecting those that affect less than five percent will require thousands of subjects.[24]

The new high-tech technology, the thousands of preliminary investigations and trials, and the many more thousands of people required for them will add considerably to the cost of drug development. As a consequence, there will be pressure put on the FDA and other regulatory agencies to allow even more corners to be cut in the research and development stage. The agencies will be asked, for example, to accept ever fewer people in all phases of trials as providing sufficient evidence to go on to the next phase, and then finally to marketing. This will result in pharmaceutical products of even more dubious value and safety than those already on the market. Finally, the drugs that do get marketed will probably be priced beyond that affordable to the vast majority of the world's population, even in First World countries.

David Horrobin has argued that genetically-targeted drugs cannot be a financially sound investment because of the complexity of the human organism and the diseases that affect it.[25]   As we shall soon see, this argument could just as well be applied to almost all other forms of gene therapy. He starts by noting that for years we have been able to identify thousands of single-gene defects but have yet to find a cure for any of them. How then is it considered likely that we will find cures for the more numerous multigenetic diseases?   But these diseases are the ones which would seem to provide the best potential market for "blockbuster drugs," those that sell in such quantity that the sales of just one or a few of them can generate a good profit for a drug company.   Almost all of the common diseases, such as diabetes, arthritis, depression, schizophrenia, heart disease, and cancer, are multigene diseases.

He does not hold out much hope of the new technology being successful even with single-gene diseases. This is because they are almost all due to loss of function of a protein and thus require an "agonist" drug, one that results in gain of a lost function. But the drug industry has not had much success in designing gain of function drugs. Such drugs must:

   1) fit well with the protein target;
   2) at the right rate of rise and fall; and
   3) limit themselves strictly to this target.

"The second and third conditions are almost impossible to achieve." If not achieved, there is a risk of ineffectiveness and of adverse side effects. A further difficulty is that most of the single-gene diseases seem to have several hundred different genetic abnormalities, each leading to a somewhat different function defect, "and a single therapeutic approach is unlikely to be applicable to all patients."

With the multigenetic common diseases, the complexity of treatment is expanded geometrically. Horrobin considers it likely that multiple-gene disorders will consist of hundreds or thousands of subdisorders, each requiring a specific and different genomics-based approach.

When one makes a sober assessment of all these problems, it becomes obvious that the required investment in this ultra-advanced strategy will most definitely be very great for any new treatment that results.   It is therefore safe to predict that the cost of treating each patient will be well beyond the limit set by Proposed Standards I and II for public funding. This, of course, is an "unmentionable" in this commercial firm-dominated research area.

Nevertheless, Horrobin is optimistic: "The likelihood is that most common diseases will be soluble and even that the solutions will be accelerated by better understanding of genomics." But the basic approach which he favors is environmentally oriented, as suggested earlier in this chapter, rather than high-tech, genomic experimentation. In his words: "We do not need any very sophisticated pharmaceuticals to perform the trick. What we do need to know is what are the environmental factors that are protecting us so successfully. And that comes down to careful clinical research."

The examples he gives are a trial to determine if a deficiency of folic acid might contribute to depression and a trial to determine if feeding a highly unsaturated fatty acid would change the lipid composition of the membrane of those who suffer from cystic fibrosis. We would note that implicit in this sort of research is the acceptance that one does not have to know exactly how something works to find out if it works. You may never find out exactly how, but you could still effect amelioration and cure. Knowing why may enable you to make even more precise and efficacious interventions, but it may also cost too much in time, effort, talent, and money to make it worthwhile to anyone other than those involved in or invested in the pursuit.

TURNING HUMANS INTO GUINEA PIGS

All of the potential forms of intervention discussed earlier are usually put under the umbrella of "gene therapy" and can be considered part of the "genomic revolution." However, this revolution did not happen overnight, though it is easy to get the impression that it did. In particular, genetic diagnosis has been around for many, many years. Long before Mendel's experiments with peas people were looking at family trees to predict certain characteristics and making conscious choices to avoid passing on of genetic defects. This is a low-tech, but efficacious, approach for many diseases. Genetic analysis of embryonic samples is more recent but has been around for at least a decade and is almost standard procedure in *in vitro* fertilization of infertile couples.

Actual "gene therapy" experiments started in 1989 with the transfer of genetically modified T cells to a patient with malignant melanoma.[26] The first allegedly successful gene therapy experiment occurred soon afterwards. In September, 1990, Asthani DeSilva, a four-year-old girl with a rare immune deficiency disease, was treated with genetically-altered white blood cells injected into her veins. The intention was to replace her defective cells with these healthy ones. Five years later, this apparently healthy and cheerful child made such an impression on the chair of the panel of the US House Science Committee, before which she appeared, that he described her as "living proof that a miracle has occurred[27]." What the chair was either unaware of or chose to ignore, as did most of the media, was that the experimental treatment was secondary to the conventional treatment that she was receiving. She had also received injections of synthetic adenosine deaminase (ADA) and, when these routine injections were withdrawn, her immune system was imperiled, despite the insertion of functioning ADA genes. Another underplayed fact was that the same treatment combination had been given to several other young children. They showed practically no evidence that the gene insertion treatment was of any value.[27,28,29] Arguably, the most unmentionable detail is the cost which was over $40,000 per month just for the conventional, synthetic ADA treatment! This is no doubt due, in part, to the fact that ADA deficiency is known to affect less than one hundred people.[16]

More recently another experiment on a another rare immune disease has received widespread publicity. The investigators claim to have enabled three infants, two with a follow-up of 11 months, to live apparently normal lives outside of a plastic bubble by virtue of genetic transfer.[30] Details as to cost and the comparative efficacy of conventional treatment are lacking, as is any broader sampling of subjects.

Similar "success stories" have become a regular feature of professional conferences, professional journals, and, naturally, of the popular media which avidly seeks out and publishes such news. In each case, the evidence is lacking that would clearly demonstrate that the genetic treatment actually works (much less of any broad or real, long-term value.[28,29] Rather, there is a rush into print, to get the good news out to the public and potential investors. Hundreds of experiments in dozens of countries have apparently led to naught in terms of actual treatment benefit.[26,31,32,33] The major problem is finding a reliable "vector" — a means of transporting the altered, healthy genes in sufficient numbers to the targeted site. But, there are also other problems. As one commentator observed: "plenty can go wrong: the newcomers might be hopelessly inept; they may be competent but find the working conditions intolerable; the natives may reject them no matter how desperately their services are needed."[34]

The other side of the coin, namely, that these experiments may have led to numerous adverse events, including deaths of the participants, has not be given the same kind of publicity. Some adverse events may not even be reported, and if they are, it is typically to an agency, such as the FDA, that does not make such reports accessible to public review.[35] "We bury our mistakes" might be their motto.

The first, and perhaps only, human death that has been attributed to this research that reached the public media was of an 18-year-old man, Jesse Gelsinger, who had a rare metabolic disorder known as OTC (deficiency of ornithine transcarbamylase). He was in good health at the commencement of the "therapy," reacted badly to the first treatment and died four days later of multiple organ failure. He, and the other 17 adults who had previously received this experimental treatment, did not really need it and could not expect to benefit from it. The curative gene was transmitted by a viral vector that was quick-acting, but whose effect was of short duration. It was really designed for another age group, that of infants born with a severe form of the condition, such that they would die within a short period of time if not helped. The treatment itself was only a stopgap to keep the infants alive long enough to find another, more effective treatment. The immune system would reject the insertion the second time around. However, infants, of course, cannot give informed consent to such experimental procedures, and it was thought that their parents, who can, might be "coerced by the disease of their child" to agree to it. Hence, it was decided to recruit adults whose disease was under control.[31,36] A question that demands an answer is whether the adult participants were fully informed in an unbiased manner before agreeing to this highly experimental intervention of no possible value to themselves.

The death of Jesse Gelsinger galvanized the press and broader investigation indicated that it was far from being a solitary incident. One syndicated columnist found "that gene therapist researchers have failed to report nearly 700 serious 'adverse events'."[37] Two other journalists noted: "Scientists and drug companies failed to notify the National Institutes of Health about six deaths that occurred in gene therapy experiments in the past 19 months, keeping details of the deaths from becoming public, according to researchers and federal officials."[38] It is still unclear whether the adverse events that occurred are due to the intervention or to other causes, such as the disease that they had. It is also not known how many other adverse events and deaths have been and are being covered up.

If all of these adverse events had been reported with as much fanfare as the purported "successes," there might now be far fewer participants willing to enter these Phase I and Phase II trials and fewer investors interested in companies that fund the research. As Nancy King, professor of social medicine at the University of North Carolina, has pointed out, calling these experiments "gene therapy trials" is a misnomer since it implies some efficacy of the treatment.[39] If a neutral, accurate description, such as "gene insertion" or "genetic intervention" trials, were used, informed consent would be facilitated on the part of potential participants. Such people now, almost automatically, assume that something therapeutic is being offered.

Obtaining informed consent must include explaining the dangers that some of the viral vectors being tried out may recombine with endogenous viruses and that germ line cells may be inadvertently modified.[40] Since germ cells are those which pass on the characteristic of parents to children, any damage to them may not manifest itself until the participants have children, at which time it may be difficult, if not impossible, to trace it to the experimental research. Still another possibility is that the material to be inserted will not be sufficiently purified, thus inadvertently introducing new diseases.

There are dangers to the general public as well. A disease which is being researched could escape from the laboratory. The procedures it has undergone could have made it even more dangerous in the meantime. To prevent this, facilities need to be built to a high specification for microbiological containment and follow rigorous safety procedures. Cryopreservation facilities need to be built for freezing and preserving the genetically modified material and expensive laboratory tests are needed to assure their quality.[26]

As illustrated by the Jesse Gelsinger case, conflict of interest is a very serious concern in the promotion of gene therapy research, indeed of the entire field of genomic research. The study that led to the death of Gelsinger, as well as other such research, was carried out by the Institute for Human Gene Therapy (IHGT) of the University of Pennsylvania. That organization is highly beholden to the Genovo Corporation and to its founder and part owner, James Wilson. He is not only director of IHGT but also has acquired federal grants that supply $5 million of its $22 million budget. In addition, Genovo and its partners, other biotech firms, have the exclusive rights to market any gene therapy "advances" developed by IHGT.[36,39]

According to Theodore Friedmann, a member of the US Recombinant DNA Advisory Committee, the informed consent process should be made more informative. Normal precautions are not enough because of the likelihood of financial conflict of interest. "There is still too ready a tendency by some in the gene therapy community to exaggerate potential benefits at the expense of full disclosure of potential risks." Accordingly, it is suggested that investigators "should disclose their direct financial ties in the informed consent process" and "those with direct financial interest in the study outcome should excuse themselves from patient selection, the informed consent process, and study direction[35]." This is seen as a minimum requirement. We might note that there is an obvious loophole: "direct financial interest." Also, the possibility of germ line damage should be included as one of the risks unless the long-term research has been done to show that it is safe. Such long-term research is not going to occur without it being forced on the companies that sponsor genetic interventions.

Friedmann further proposes tightening the reporting of adverse events. Investigators in the USA are required to report "serious, unexpected or related" events to the FDA within 15 days. However, "serious, unexpected or related" are terms open to interpretation, and hence subject to biases by the investigators and study sponsors. Another writer notes that it is not just investigators (or outside sponsors) that may have conflicts of interests, but also the institute itself.[41] This is obviously true of the institute at the University of Pennsylvania in the Jesse Gelsinger case. In today's university-industry "co-operative climate," stringent guidelines need to be applied also to university projects.

Subsequent to the disclosure of the adverse events mentioned above, several calls were made for stricter guidelines and more public disclosure as a means of controlling the dominant role of free enterprise in this field. The necessity for this comes not only from possible conflict of interest but also from the great cost of this research combined with poor prospects of success. Just production and testing of a single vector for introducing healthy genes to replace defective ones exceeds several hundred thousand dollars.[35] And, to date, no reliable vector has been identified.[40] A complicating factor is that many diseases have many different mutations. For example, cystic fibrosis, a favorite target of genetic intervention research since 1993 because it is the most common single-gene defect, has around 700 mutations.[42,43] If a treatment is found that works for one mutation, there is no guarantee that it or something similar, will work for any other mutation. This does not mean that vectors will not be found which work for some diseases and for some of those who suffer from them. All this, plus the cost for the array of the very expensive high-tech equipment which are typically required, makes genetic research the most expensive technology of all of modern medicine. This creates the very real possibility that these serious difficulties of the whole enterprise will make it highly tempting for corners to be cut in the safety department. This can occur in three key areas: proceeding to clinical trials prematurely, failing to obtain informed consent in a completely honest fashion, and exposing the public to potential dangers.

The other obvious area where guidelines are needed, such as those of the Proposed Standards VIII to XIII, is in the area of publication. As of now, without these conflict of interest standards, an enormous propaganda campaign is in full swing. Ironically, the clearest description of this that we have read is by two authors, one of whom is a former president of the Pharmaceutical Research Institute of Bristol-Myers Squibb. They state[41]:

> *Since the inception of its clinical trials a decade ago, gene therapy's leading proponents have given the field a continuous positive 'spin' that is unusual for most medical research. Yet, despite repeated claims of benefit or even cure, no single unequivocal instance of clinical efficacy exists in the hundreds of gene therapy trials.*

One can understand the enthusiasm of those who believe we are on the verge of discovering the basic secrets of life and turning this knowledge into cures which seem to border on the miraculous, but, in today's financial climate, such unremitting promotion of a high-tech industry more closely resembles ads by used car dealers than scientific journalism.

GENETIC ENHANCEMENT

There is one last set of promises that warrant some attention: those that are directed, not at cure or alleviation of a disease or other crippling condition, but rather at improving the lot of normal, healthy individuals. It is cosmetic surgery at the genetic level: shortness and baldness are among the targets as is, in women, an undesirable shape. There is, of course, a gulf between finding genes that contribute to these conditions and actually doing something about it. But, if the market is thought to be there, the temptation is strong to pursue this line of research. The cost of such "cures" will certainly be in the gazillion dollar range.

Let us imagine for a moment that genetic treatments become widely available for people who are dissatisfied with their height, baldness, or shape. While this may be excellent for the self-image of the person "cured," it creates on a society level as many problems as it solves. This is because those not given the treatment will now feel even more disadvantaged as their numbers will have noticeably shrunk.

What is more worrisome yet is the research on how to slow down or halt the aging process. The age issue concerns everyone, and it is conceivable that those who are getting older, and not gracefully so, and those who simply want to remain "forever young" will join together and demand public funding of research in this area. Such demands were fed by a recent article that favorably reported on experiments which indicated that insertion of certain genes extends the lives of mice.[44] The question of what would happen to our society, indeed to our planet, if we were to be successful in pursuit of this path is not likely to be raised in research protocols or in the approval process, or, if raised, to be more than myopically answered.

CONCLUDING REMARKS

We can summarize this chapter with a question: What would our world be like if we didn't pursue the yellow brick road that leads us to the Kingdom of Genetic Knowledge? Would we be worse off than we are now, or better off, or some of both? If the goal is to improve the health of human beings in general, and not just small groupings of them, then the answer is clear. As Richard Powers[45], author of *Gain*, puts it:

> *As we pursue ever more exotic biological techniques, we lag ever further behind in putting existing medical technology to proper use. The health benefits deriving from stem cell research are likely to be arcane and expensive, and nowhere near as consequential to world health as, say, the application of existing low-tech treatments for malnutrition and infant diarrhea.*

What he says in regard to stem cell research applies at least as well to research on high-tech genomic intervention. We simply cannot pursue everything that interests us, neither as individuals nor as societies. As individuals we have to ask how much time, energy, and money the pursuit is likely to require in order to realize any benefits, or is it a pursuit that is worth it in itself, as the best ones are.

As societies, we need to ask what impact is it likely to have on those around us, and what activities would be interfered with or would have to be relinquished. Perhaps the most vital question to pose is the ethical one: Is it an honorable pursuit or is it something that doesn't feel quite right, despite its appeal? When individuals do not follow their conscience, they reduce the basic control they have over what they become. Now societies don't really have consciences, but they consist of people who do. By their behavior they contribute to the formation of implicit guidelines which steer our society. In the field of medicine it is all too often the guideline of "I demand the best, no matter what it may cost (others)." And "the best" is whatever people have been led to think is best by the heavily commercialized popular (and professional) media. It is possible to change this guideline, and, as this book argues, it is essential to do so if we are to have anything left over for social justice and environmentalism or for other worthy causes.

As Daniel Callahan notes: "The very nature of medical progress is to pull to itself many more resources than can be of genuine benefit to many individuals, and much, much more than can be socially justifiable for the common good."[46] High-tech medical research is a ravenous creature whose appetite not only is never satisfied, but grows by feeding it. It can resemble a cancer in our society. This book has attempted to demonstrate that fact and has crafted some guidelines which, if followed, would starve the cancerous growth without harming the body of sound medical research and practice.

The latest, most virulent metastasized outbreak of this cancer is genomic research. It is both tremendously demanding of resources and obviously capable of swallowing everything fed it in terms of money and other resources. It is, nevertheless, very appealing, because of the glorious mantle in which it is draped. As two commentators conclude in a recent article in the *New England Journal of Medicine*[47]:

> *Although we do not contend that the genetic mantle is as imperceptible as the emperor's new clothes were, it is not made of the silks and ermines that some claim it to be. Those who make medical and science policies in the next decade would do well to see beyond the hype.*

We have gone about the task of examining the worth of this enterprise by removing its mantle. We have shown its lack of substance and noted the incredible start-up investment it has taken to get to this point of practically zero achievement. Given this, would it truly be right for us to make this a higher priority than almost any other pursuit in medicine? Or is this a case of demand the best, even it is only the promise of the best, regardless what it costs (others)"?

We should not be surprised that these questions are seldom posed. We have been too inundated with hyperbole over advances in knowledge that are being made based on having largely "mapped" the genome of humans as well as that of several other creatures. Politicians and other prominent figures have augmented this message with their uncritical, populist statements and generous funding.

A major reason why attempts to translate gene therapy research into medical practice are likely, by their very nature, to be unethical is that the whole field may be doomed because of its astronomical complexity. Existing information already constitutes a state of extreme information overload. This problem is becoming rapidly more overwhelming. First, researchers are continuing at breakneck speed to map more and more of the thousands of genes of interest. As yet, we have not even done more than scratch the surface of the human genome. On top of this, each gene may be either turned on or off, and this adds an additional layer of extreme complexity. And for good measure, we should not forget the almost infinite number of possible mutations. Scientists admit this task is daunting, but they do not recognize that to pursue the basically impractical and highly expensive at the cost of practical pursuits is unethical.

Horrobin[25] touched on the impracticability of this issue in his discussion of the prospects for developing profitable, genetically-targeted drugs, and it is worth repeating here:

> *The implications of a successful genomics program are only marginally less devastating to the current pharmaceutical industry than would be a total failure of that program. . . If a*

> *disease such as cystic fibrosis, due to a single gene, is now seen to be made up of hundreds of different specific genetic abnormalities, the likelihood is that multiple-gene disorders will actually consist of hundreds of thousands of subdisorders, each with a specific and different genomics-based approach. . .But this all depends on the success of the genomics-based therapeutic program. Neither industry executives nor government regulators should lose much sleep; failure is a much more likely outcome.*

One would think this would become self-evident to the industry at some point and the market would be the correcting influence, as Novartis has shown with its cutback of its investment in developing organs for transplantation from genetically-humanized pigs.[48] But in today's world this is not always true, as demonstrated by the profits being made by those who offer DNA chip testing. These computer chips are worse than useless for the great majority of diseases because they don't, and cannot, give precise information about what will happen to those who are found to have "disease genes." The most they are good for is as gifts for the very rich, who will use them as a conversation piece, rather like many people do with predictions from horoscopes. Taken seriously, they would only confuse and mislead. The likely value of advice that patients will receive is indicated by a survey done by the Human Genome project: only 54 percent of the physicians who responded had even one course in basic genetics.[49] Compounding this, some physicians may be influenced by their financial ties to the companies that provide the tests.[50]

As long as someone can turn a short-term profit, then information, gadgetry, products and procedures will be marketed, and marketed aggressively, almost regardless of worth. Only if they can be shown to lead to near-future, provable harm, will they be withdrawn. Actual usefulness is not the typical criterion in much, if not most, of high-tech medical practice, and research that looks to produce something saleable is more important than research that will lead to something clearly of value. Assessment of long-term negative effects, such as germ line damage, are seldom, if ever, part of research protocols. And short-term investors in company stocks are primarily, if not exclusively, interested in companies whose research regularly leads to public announcements of "breakthroughs." They do not plan to stick around to see if any discoveries actually result in anything. For example, shares in Affymetrix, the pioneering company in DNA diagnostic chips, quintupled in 1998.[51] And Celera, the privately owned company that mapped the human genome, charges companies $5 million to $15 million per year for access to the data.[52]

Genomics has created a scientific Alice in Wonderland world: humans are used as guinea pigs while pigs are humanized!

There are, however, a few bright spots on the horizon. We have mentioned some before, such as the increased awareness by editors of professional journals of the dangers posed to the publication process by financial conflicts of interest of authors and peer reviewers. Also, there is increased awareness by the relevant parts of the medical industry that there are legal risks for them in this new field. Merck, a pharmaceutical giant, refused to allow use of its patented process for development of a safer virus vector for fear that it would not turn out to be so safe, and, as a result, Merck would incur at least partial liability.[53] As a result of a growing appreciation of the hazards of genetic testing, the US Health and Human Services Secretary is considering what needs to be done to ensure the quality of such tests, being that the FDA says it lacks the required resources.[12]

Perhaps the most positive sign of a change to more realistic assessment of what can be realized is the establishment of a federal Office for Human Research Protection in the USA and the professed policy of its incoming head, Greg Koski. He is said to support the idea that "scientists should have no financial ties to companies whose policies they are testing."[54] He responded to the contention of some critics that "there are certain financial conflicts of interest that cannot be avoided" by stating, "I believe they probably should be avoided in most instances." With respect to the failure of the policy of relying on academia to police itself, he noted that academic-industry ties "have gotten completely out of control." Showing much the same mind-set the board of directors of the American Society of Gene Therapy declared in April, 2000, that clinical researchers should have no "equity, stock options, or similar arrangements" with companies sponsoring trials. Alas, it would be naive to believe that this will stop the myriad of ways in which sponsors can affect the designing, execution, analysis, and reporting of trial results, but it is certainly a start.

References

[1] Temple NJ, Burkitt DB (1991). The war on cancer – failure of therapy and research. *J R Soc Med* 84: 95-98.

[2] Temple NJ (1985). Simplicity – the key to fruitful medical research. *Med Hypotheses* 17: 139-45.

[3] Temple NJ (1994). Medical research. A complex problem. In: Temple NJ, Burkitt DB, eds. *Western diseases: their dietary prevention and reversibility.* Totowa, NJ: Humana Press: 419-36.

[4] Lichtenstein P, Holm NV. et al. (2000). Environmental and heritable factors in the causation of cancer. *N Eng J Med* 343: 78-85.

[5] Hoover RN (2000). Cancer – nature, nurture, or both. *N Engl J Med* 343: 135-36.

[6] Yamey G (2000). Scientists unveil first draft of human genome. *BMJ* 321: 7.

[7] Rehmann-Sutter C (September 28, 2000). Liefert Genom wirklich die Rohdaten für "den Menschen"? *Basler Zeitung*: 3.

[8] Brown K (July, 2000). The human genome business today. *Sci Amer*: 50-55.

[9] Rusconi S (December 1, 1999). Gentherapie-Forscher: verkannte Helden oder Roulettespieler? *Neue Zürcher Zeitung*: 77.

[10] Marshall E (1995). Gene therapy's growing pains. *Science* 269:1050-55.

[11] Steinberg D (2000). DNA chips. *The Scientist* 14: 1, 12-13.

[12] Weiss R (July 2, 1999). Mistakes in genetic testing show need for controls. *International Herald Tribune*: 2.

[13] Yan H, Kinzler K W, & Vogelstein B (2000). Genetic testing – present and future. *Science* 289: 1890-92.

[14] Wormer VH (2000). Orakelsprüche aus dem Erbgut. *Pressespiegel: Gentechnologie* 40: 34.

[15] Suzuki DT, Knudtson P (1989). *Genetics: The clash between the new genetics and human values.* Cambridge, MA: Harvard University Press.

[16] Colen BD (1986). *Hard choices: mixed blessings of modern medical technology.* New York: G. P. Putman's Sons.

[17] Bobrow M, Grimbaldeston AH (2000). Medical genetics, the human genome project and public health. *J Epidimiol Community Health* 54: 645-49.

[18] Asraf H (2000). Less counseling needed for genetic testing of colorectal cancer. *Lancet* 355: 2141.

[19] Clarfield AM (1999). Genetic testing for Alzheimer disease. *N Engl J Med* 341: 1160-61.

[20] Stephenson J (1994). Alzheimer's update: a mixed blessing. *Harvard Health Letter*: 20: 1-3.

[21] Council on Ethical and Judicial Affairs, American Medical Association (1991). Use of genetic testing by employers. *JAMA* 266: 1827-30.

[22] Draper E (July-August, 1992). Genetic secrets: social issues of medical screening in a genetic age. *Hastings Center Report* (Special Supplement): S15-18.

[23] Weatherall D (1995). *Science and the quiet art.* New York: W. W. Norton and Company.

[24] Bonn D (1999). Early results on cataloguing SNPs suggests task bigger than first thought. *Lancet* 354: 49.

[25] Horrobin DF (2000). Innovation in the pharmaceutical industry. *J R Soc Med* 93: 341-45.

[26] Russel SJ (2000). Gene therapy. *BMJ* 315: 1289-92.

[27] Marshall E (1995). Gene therapy's growing pains. *Science* 269:1050-55.

[28] Kohn DB, Hershfield MS, et al. (1998). T lymphocytes with a normal ADA gene accumulate after transplantation of transduced autologous umbilical cord blood CD34+ cells in ADA-deficient SCID neonates. *Nature Medicine* 14: 775-80.

[29] Calvazzana-Calvo M, Hacein-Bey S, et al. (2000). *Science* 288: 669-72.

[30] Gene therapy: when and for what? (1995). *Lancet* 345: 739-40.

[31] Miller HI (February 7, 2000). Gene therapy's trials and tribulations. *The Scientist* 14: 16.

[32] Rosenberg LE, Schechter AN (2000). Gene therapist, heal yourself. *Science* 287: 1751.

[33] Lennard AL, Jackson GH (2000). Stem cell transplantation. *BMJ* 321: 433-37.

[34] Thomas P (1992). New hope for old diseases. *Harvard Health Letter* 17: 1-4.

[35] Friedmann T (2000). Principles for human gene therapy studies. *Science* 287: 2163, 2165.

[36] Marshall E (2000). Gene therapy on trial. *Science* 288: 951-57.

[37] Goodman E (February 17, 2000). A medical promised land strewn with dangers. *International Herald Tribune*: 11.

[38] Nelson D, Weiss R (November 4, 1999). 6 deaths in gene therapy concealed. *International Herald Tribune*: 2.

[39] Halim NS (2000). Gene therapy institute faces uphill battle. *The Scientist* 14: 1,12.

[40] Mitchell P (1998). Vector problems still thwart gene-therapy promise. *Lancet* 351: 346.

[41] Rosenberg LE, Schechter AN (2000). Gene therapist, heal thyself. *Science* 287: 1751.

[42] Associated Press (April 20, 1993). Gene transfer is tried to cure cystic fibrosis. *Register-Guard*, Eugene OR: 7A.

[43] Holmes LB (1998). Screening for cystic fibrosis. *JAMA* 279: 1068-69.

[44] Wade N (September 28, 2000). Searching for the genes that control aging. *International Herald Tribune*: 10.

[45] Powers R (November 20, 1998). All this biotechnology is scary. *International Herald Tribune*: 12.

[46] Silverman WA (1998). *Where's the evidence?* New York: Oxford University Press: 71.

[47] Holtzman NA, Marteau TM (2000). Will genetics revolutionize medicine? *N Engl J Med* 343: 141-44.

[48] Novartis fährt Xeno-Forschung zurück (September 27, 2000). *Basler Zeitung*. Basel, Switzerland: 17.

[49] The Council on Ethical and Judicial Affairs, American Medical Association (July-August, 1998). Multiplex genetic testing. *Hasting Center Report*: 15-21.

[50] Silverman PH (May-June, 1995). Commerce and genetic diagnostics. *Hasting Center Report* (Special Supplement): S15-S17.

[51] Fisher LM (December 23, 1999). DNA analysis gets personal. *International Herald Tribune*: 8.

[52] Friend T (June 23, 2000). Genome project completes sequence. *USA Today*: 1A-2A.

[53] Smaglik P (2000). Merck blocks "safer" gene therapy trials. *Nature* 403: 817.

[54] Agnew B (2000). Financial conflicts get more scrutiny in clinical trials. *Science* 289: 1266-67.

Chapter Eleven

Disease Prevention: The Low-Tech, Low-Cost Road Less Travelled

Norman J. Temple

"On the big issues the experts are very rarely right." Peter Wright in Spycatcher (1987)

In the several preceding chapters we have discussed how a dominant theme of much medical research is the search for new treatments. Typically, when new treatments are developed, they are high-tech and inevitably expensive, often to the extent that they are unaffordable for many people, even in First World countries. This problem is frequently compounded by a second problem: these new treatments are often put into practice without having to meet strict standards of efficacy, and, in many cases can actually result in more harm than good. A major reason for these problems is the profit motive: increasingly researchers and physicians profit financially from their relationship with commercial firms and this influences how research is carried out and how the results are interpreted and disseminated. Overall, the degree of success of modern medicine has been a good deal less than the spokespeople for medicine claim or that they routinely promise is just around the corner.

In this chapter we explore an alternative strategy. Over the last quarter century a vast amount of evidence has accumulated demonstrating that the key determinant of the major diseases that afflict Western societies is lifestyle. The obvious inference from this is that these diseases are preventable. This knowledge can be translated into effective action for disease prevention at the population level. This strategy potentially requires far less resources to accomplish far more than does the search for and utilization of new high-tech treatments.

A strategy focused on prevention has another outstanding advantage. Even where a disease can be successfully treated, it is self-evidently better to prevent that disease, or at least to postpone it until later in life. Using the

169

A. Thompson and N.J. Temple (eds.), Ethics, Medical Research, and Medicine, 169–187.
© 2001 *Kluwer Academic Publishers. Printed in the Netherlands.*

measure of Quality-Adjusted Life Years, the measure advocated in chapter three, will inevitably show that disease prevention is highly effective.

History teaches us the value of prevention. The greatest achievement of biomedical science during the past 150 years was the conquest of many infectious diseases. The lion's share of credit for this belongs to primary prevention, especially the widespread adoption of hygiene. Medical treatment, by contrast, played a fairly minor role. There is no reason why a prevention strategy cannot be made to repeat this great success story, this time against chronic diseases.

The potential impact of a preventive approach is dramatically illustrated by the following examples:

- Selenium is a mineral which epidemiological evidence has indicated is protective against cancer. As a test of this a randomized intervention trial was conducted in which subjects were given either placebo or a supplement of selenium. During the six years of the study cancer mortality fell by half.[1]

- A study on subjects recovering from heart disease was carried out in Lyon, France. Subjects were given either a regular heart diet or one modified to resemble a Mediterranean diet. In particular, it was rich in omega-3 fatty acids that were provided by canola oil. These fats are similar to the fats found in fatty fish. After four years, risk of death from both heart disease and cancer each fell by more than half.[2,3] (Although the intervention was used as a therapy, the findings are equally relevant to primary prevention.)

- A long-term study was carried out on 84,000 American nurses. The investigators estimated that the risk of coronary disease in the three percent with the healthiest lifestyle was six times lower than in the rest of the nurses.[4]

The three leading aspects of lifestyle involved in causing and preventing the chronic diseases are nutrition, smoking, and, to a lesser extent, exercise. Many people assumed that after this information was discovered, the next step was to disseminate this information to the public and exhort lifestyle changes. This, hopefully, would bring about the necessary changes. But despite countless television programs and articles in the mass media it has proven extremely difficult to translate this knowledge into changes in behavior at the population level. Certainly, millions have listened to the message and changed their lifestyles but the degree of success has been far less than what has been hoped for.

The following surveys' findings illustrate the gulf that separates hope from reality:

- The prevalence of obesity jumped by about seven percent in American adults between 1976-80 and 1988-94.[5] Between 1991 and 1998 the weight of the average American adult rose by more than three kilograms.[6] Similar trends have been reported from other Western countries.[7]

- Although consumption of fruit and vegetables has increased in the USA since the 1970s, nevertheless, only around 22 percent of Americans consume the recommended five or more servings per day of these foods.[8] Moreover, on any given day half of Americans eat no fruit.[9]

- While millions have taken up exercise, far greater numbers have been left behind. For instance, among middle-aged adults in England no more than one half of men and one quarter of women engage in at least moderate exercise, such as a brisk walk for at least 30 minutes on five or more days each week.[10] About one third of American adults achieve this level of exercise[11], while another third report no leisure time exercise.[12]

HEALTH PROMOTION CAMPAIGNS

Starting in the 1970s various intervention projects have been carried out with the aim of encouraging people to lead a healthier lifestyle and thereby prevent disease. The major aim has generally been the prevention of coronary heart disease (CHD). Accordingly, interventions have most often been directed at blood cholesterol, blood pressure, weight control, exercise, and smoking. These interventions are reviewed here and conclusions drawn as to how medicine can more effectively prevent disease.

Community-based campaigns

Various intervention campaigns have targeted entire communities using a variety of approaches such as presentations in schools, displays in supermarkets, and delivering information through the mass media. The results have been mixed.

During the 1980s three large-scale projects were carried out in the USA. Each program lasted five to eight years and aimed to persuade people to exercise, to cut smoking rates, and to lower elevated levels of blood cholesterol, blood pressure, and weight. The three programs succeeded in implementing a wide range of interventions and involving large numbers of participants.

The Stanford Five-City Project was carried out in California.[13]   Two intervention cities received health education via TV, radio, newspapers, other mass-distributed print media, as well as by direct education and through schools.   On average each adult received 26 hours of education. This was achieved at a cost of four dollars per person per year, which is about 800 times less than total health-care costs.   The Minnesota Heart Health Program included three intervention cities and three control cities in the Upper Midwest.[14]   The third project was the Pawtucket Heart Health Program.[15]   Here, the population of Pawtucket, Rhode Island, received intensive education at the grass roots level: schools, local government, community organizations, supermarkets, and so forth. The media were not involved.

The results of the three studies were combined, thereby giving a sample size of 12 cities.[16]   Considering the great effort put into these intervention projects, the results were disappointing.   Improvements in blood pressure, blood cholesterol, weight, and smoking were of very low magnitude and were not statistically significant; there was no change in the estimated risk of CHD.   A similar lack of success was also reported in two more recent community projects.[17,18]

One possibility that could explain these discouraging results is that the interventions took place at a time when there were already trends towards a healthier lifestyle and a fall in the incidence of CHD.   Most Americans had already heard the "message" and those who were so inclined had to some extent already changed their ways.   It may be that a health promotion campaign is unlikely to succeed if it takes place against a background of improving lifestyles.

The best known example of a successful community intervention for the prevention of CHD was carried out in North Karelia.[19]   This region of eastern Finland had an exceptionally high rate of the disease.   The intervention, which was based on a nutrition education campaign, began in 1972 at which time few people were aware of how lifestyle changes could reduce the risk of CHD.   The people of North Karelia responded well to the campaign and CHD rates fell sharply over the next few years.   In response to this the intensive educational campaign was extended to the rest of Finland with a resulting drop in CHD rates.[20]

A lesser degree of success was achieved in two other European studies. The German Cardiovascular Prevention Study resembled the American community studies in that a variety of methods were used to encourage a healthier lifestyle.[21]   It was carried out in the former West Germany from about 1985 to 1992 when there was no particular favorable trend in risk factors. The intervention led to a small decrease in blood pressure and serum cholesterol (about two percent) and a seven percent fall in smoking, but had no effect on weight. Action Heart was a community-based health promotion campaign conducted in Rotherham, England, over a four-year period.[22] Positive changes were recorded in some parameters—seven percent fewer people smoked and nine percent more drank low-fat milk—but there was no change in exercise habits, obesity, or consumption of wholemeal bread.

Two recent intervention projects represent a radical departure from the strategy used in the above studies. Rather than aiming to simultaneously improve several aspects of lifestyle, the focus was on just one change. The studies used paid advertising as the major educational tool rather than a variety of tools.

The 1% Or Less campaign used paid advertising in the media as the sole component of the intervention.[23] The objective was to persuade the population of a city in West Virginia to switch from whole milk to low-fat milk (1% or less). Despite a budget of under a dollar per person, low-fat milk sales, as a proportion of total milk sales, increased from 29 percent to 46 percent within just a few weeks. The second project was carried out in the State of Victoria, Australia, from 1992 to 1995 and aimed to increase consumption of fruit and vegetables.[24] Paid advertising was a major component. Consumption increased by 11 percent for fruit and by 17 percent for vegetables.

While the results are highly variable and often disappointing, these groundbreaking approaches to persuading whole communities to improve their lifestyles indicate that educational approaches at the community level can potentially prevent much disease.

Worksite health promotion

Many attempts have been made to bring work promotion to the worksite. Employers, no doubt, are motivated by the hope that if the workers become healthier they will also be more productive and costs associated with sickness will be reduced.

The following examples are illustrative of this approach. The Treatwell program in New England encouraged employees to reduce their fat intake and to increase their intake of fiber.[25] A modest decrease in fat intake was observed (three percent) but with no change in fiber. In a development of this program employees and their families were encouraged to increase their intake of fruit and vegetables; a rise of 19 percent was achieved.[26] A similar project in Minnesota offered employees weight control and smoking cessation programs.[27] As is often the case the degree of success was much less than had been hoped for: compared with control worksites, body weight did not change but the prevalence of smoking was reduced by two percent.

Health promotion as a medical intervention

An obvious place to conduct health promotion is the doctor's office. After all, people generally listen to advice given by their doctor or other health professional. Several such interventions have been carried out.

Two randomized trials were carried out in Britain during the early 1990s with the goal of reducing risk of cardiovascular disease by lifestyle intervention. The interventions were done in the offices of family physicians, with the health advice being given by nurses. The OXCHECK study reported no significant effect on smoking or excessive alcohol intake but did observe small significant improvements in exercise participation, weight, dietary intake of saturated fat, and serum cholesterol.[28,29] The Family Heart Study reported that the estimated risk of CHD was reduced by 12 percent.[30] Thus, despite intensive efforts, the interventions achieved only modest changes.

A meta-analysis was carried out on 17 randomized controlled intervention trials where dietary advice was given to adults.[31] The interventions were mostly done in a medical setting on subjects who had risk factors for disease (mostly hypertension, hypercholesterolemia, or were at risk of breast cancer). Over the course of nine to 18 months of follow-up there were small decreases in serum cholesterol and blood pressure, and this lowered the estimated risk of CHD by 14 percent.

To a considerable extent the above studies were on subjects at above average risk of CHD. This is probably the most cost-effective form of intervention as, first, subjects are more likely than the average person to follow the advice and, second, a behavior change is more likely to prevent a case of CHD in a high-risk subject than in a low-risk subject.[32] The following Swedish study is an example of focusing on subjects at relatively high risk of cardiovascular disease[33] Subjects were given either simple advice from their physician or intensive advice (five 90-minute sessions plus an all-day session). The intensive advice had a modest impact; it reduced the estimated risk of CHD by some six percent.

While the high-risk approach is more cost-effective than giving advice to the entire population, it does have a major deficiency. As pointed out by Rose[34] a majority of future cases of CHD are excluded. This is because the 15 percent of men at "high risk" of CHD account for only 32 percent of cases. It follows, therefore, that to achieve a substantial drop in the incidence of CHD it is necessary to target the entire population. The same principle applies to other chronic diseases such as cancer and stroke. In other words, we must recognize that it the population as a whole that is at risk and in need of a healthier diet and lifestyle.

The impact of health promotion

Results of attempts to educate the public to the necessity of lifestyle change have been quite variable: negligible changes in some studies but impressive changes in others. The batting average suggests that risk factors move in the right direction by typically a few percent and this would be expected to cut the risk of CHD by five to 15 percent. It must be emphasized at this point that the percentage changes in disease risk discussed here are relative rather than absolute changes. For reasons discussed in chapter four, absolute change is the preferred form of presenting such data as relative change can be misleading. Nevertheless, as CHD accounts for about one third of all deaths, a decrease in the risk of CHD of five to 15 percent is self-evidently a major public health achievement.

We need to make an objective evaluation of this level of change. It certainly constitutes an important step in the right direction. But at the same time most people are little affected. It follows, therefore, that attempts to make deep cuts in the levels of such diseases as cardiovascular disease and cancer by appealing to people to modify their lifestyles are therefore unlikely to succeed. Health promotion, whether through the media, in the community, at the worksite, or in the physician's office, is valuable as far as it goes but has a strictly limited impact.

However, even the fairly small changes brought about by health promotion can make valuable contributions to public health which fully justifies the time and effort involved. For instance, Jeffery, et al.[27] concluded that a smoking cessation program at a worksite costs about $100 to $200 per smoker who quits. Similarly, Action Heart estimated that the cost per year of life gained was a mere 31 British pounds.[22] This indicates that to generate one year of life using health promotion costs less than $50. By contrast the comparable cost using statin drugs is at least $50,000 (chapter seven). These numbers eloquently speak for themselves.

Let us return to the major theme of this book: making medical research truly of value. There is a pressing need for studies to determine why different health promotion projects have achieved such varying levels of success. Perhaps the focus should be on one lifestyle change rather than many. Perhaps the most cost-effective means to utilize scarce resources is paid advertising.

GOVERNMENT POLICY

Why do most studies show a rather low degree of response to health education? In retrospect it is somewhat naive to expect people to change the habits of a lifetime from interventions that merely exhort the individual to lead a healthier lifestyle. There are many factors that determine our behavior. For instance, fashion and peer pressure strongly influence our receptiveness to new ideas. Our choices at the store are strongly influenced by both price and the advertising to which we are perpetually bombarded.

But this does not mean that we should be resigned to the limited effectiveness of the type of health promotion interventions described earlier. Rather, we must learn lessons and formulate a new strategy. A truly effective strategy must be based on the reasons that people make choices. What this translates to is that the central component of new interventions will be policy changes by governments.

The effect of price on sales

Governments have the power to pass legislation and to manipulate prices using taxation and subsidies. These government powers have tremendous potential for influencing health behavior. The most convincing evidence demonstrating this comes from studies on smoking.

There is no doubt that health education has been of huge importance in reducing the prevalence of smoking. This is convincingly shown by the 50 percent fall since the 1960s in the proportion of men who smoke. But this still leaves every third or fourth adult in most Western countries as die-hard smokers.

The method of proven effectiveness to bring down smoking rates is an increase in price.[35] Smoking shows what economists refer to as "price elasticity": a ten percent increase in price reduces smoking by about five percent, especially among the lower socioeconomic groups.[36] A rise in price has more impact on smoking than does education or media campaigns.[37]

Canada provides the clearest illustration of this. During the 1980s the price of cigarettes doubled in that country and at the same time smoking rates among young adults fell by half. However, large-scale smuggling took place during the early 1990s (engineered in part by the tobacco companies). In response to this the tax, and hence the price, of cigarettes was cut with the predictable result that the fall in smoking rates among young adults promptly went into reverse.[38]

There is little doubt, then, that price rises are a far more effective and reliable means to bring about decreases in smoking prevalence than are health promotion interventions.

Studies of the relationship between the price of alcohol and consumption reveal a similar price elasticity: a price rise of ten percent causes a decrease in consumption of between three and eight percent.[39]

The lesson we learn from cigarettes and alcohol is also true for food. Every supermarket manager knows that in order to quickly sell fruit that is becoming overripe, it is necessary to lower the price. From this we can make a critically important inference: **the judicious use of taxes and subsidies are a sure means to persuade people to increase consumption of fruit, vegetables, and whole-grain cereals, while lowering consumption of less healthy choices such as fat-rich food**. This assertion is the basis of the blueprint for action suggested here. In actuality, this concept has been around for a number of years. The World Health Organization made a similar recommendation at the Adelaide Conference in 1988: "Taxation and subsidies should discriminate in favor of easy access for all to healthy food and improved diet."[40]

Jeffery and colleagues in the USA have carried out studies to investigate the effectiveness of this approach. In one study at a worksite the price of low-fat snacks sold in vending machines was halved. As a result sales of these foods jumped from 26 percent of total sales before intervention to 46 percent after.[41] In another intervention, which was done in a worksite cafeteria, they succeeded in trebling sales of fruit and salad items by halving the price while also widening the choices that were available.[42] A similar study was conducted in a high school cafeteria. The price of fruit, carrots, and salads was halved, resulting in a fourfold increase in sales of fruit, a twofold increase for carrots, and a slight increase for salads.[43] What these studies graphically reveal is the potential of policy interventions, especially of low prices, to redirect food choices towards healthy foods.

Advertising, marketing, and labeling of food

Food advertising appears to be another factor that exerts a major influence on people's diets.[44] After all, the fact that commercial enterprises, large and small, spend so lavishly on advertising is eloquent testimony as to its effectiveness. It is scarcely surprising that health promotion campaigns achieve such poor levels of success when they must compete against ubiquitous advertising of unhealthy food choices. For instance, the annual promotion costs for soft drinks in the USA is up to $116m and for McDonald's is just over a billion dollars.[45] This type of spending dwarfs the million dollars spent annually by the National Cancer Institute on the education component of its 5-a-Day campaign to promote fruit and vegetable consumption.

Food advertisers spare no effort to win over the hearts and mouths of children to junk food. An American study of advertisements appearing on Saturday morning TV, a peak viewing time for children, found that 44 percent were for fats, oils, and sugar, 23 percent were for highly-sugared cereals, and 11 percent were for fast-food restaurants.[46] By contrast, the percentage devoted to fruit and vegetables was zero. The authors concluded that: "The diet that is presented on Saturday morning television is the antithesis of what is recommended for healthful eating for children." Much the same situation prevails in Canada.[47]

The marketing strategy of the food industry extends well beyond advertising. For instance, because there is a growing market for low-fat foods, manufacturers sell foods with less fat, but the missing fat often reappears in foods which may be little more than concoctions of fat, sugar, and salt.[48] The food industry promotes high-fat food because it is so profitable.[49] This problem is compounded by the fact that food labeling is confusing to most consumers; even if they want low-fat foods, the labels do not facilitate making the right choices. This is truer of Britain than of the USA. The system is, in theory, based on "consumer choice" but, in reality, choices become largely uninformed ones.

It is apparent, therefore, that much progress could be made towards improving dietary patterns by curtailing the excesses of the advertising industry and by ensuring that all food, including fresh meat and food sold in restaurants and convenience stores, is clearly labeled.

The necessity for public health policies

A strong case can be made, therefore, that desirable changes in eating patterns will only be achieved when governments implement public health policies in such areas as food prices, food advertising, and labeling. The following are specific suggestions formulated by Marion Nestle of New York University as to how this might be done so as to encourage diets higher in fruit and vegetables and lower in fat[50]:

1. By the redirection of subsidies, better labeling, and perhaps even taxation, the sale of low-fat types of meat and milk could be encouraged over high-fat types.
2. Schools could be pressured to sell healthier food while restricting the sale of junk food. Such an approach is equally applicable to other institutions under government control, such as the military, prisons, and cafeterias in government offices and hospitals.

3. Restrictions should be placed on the advertising of unhealthy food products. This is of especial importance for TV advertising directed at children.

This strategy can be applied to other areas of lifestyle, especially to smoking. Similarly, policy initiatives can be used to encourage more people to exercise. Many people are dissuaded from taking exercise because of the various barriers that exist, such as a lack of appropriate facilities and roads that are too dangerous for bikes. Here government policies could directly tackle these barriers.

Given the dismal record of both health education and of therapeutic medicine in their dealings with obesity, it is scarcely surprising that a public health policy approach has been suggested several times as a more effective means to lower the prevalence of this condition. For example, Robert Jeffery[51] of the University of Minnesota School of Public Health argued that: "I believe that it is time to think about alternatives to the traditional individual-focused strategies for obesity control. I believe we should also view our food supply as a potential environmental hazard that promotes obesity and to consider public health policy strategies for improving it." James[49] and later Nestle and Jacobson[52] also made proposals for how public health policies could be used to help combat obesity.

The rationale for a public health policy approach was well put by Henry Blackburn[53] of the University of Minnesota:

> *...even the newer community-based lifestyle strategies continue to assign much of the burden of change to the individual. A shift of focus to reducing, by policy change, many widespread practices that are life-threatening, while enhancing life-supportive practices, should redirect the currently misplaced emphasis on achieving 'responsible' behavior and its purported difficulty. For example, local communities may more appropriately be considered to have a 'youth tobacco access problem,' approachable in part by regulation, than a 'youth smoking problem,' approachable mainly by education. Policy interventions may also be designed to . . . make preventive practice more economical, as well as to encourage the development of more healthy products by industry. They may be a partial answer to another major paradox: while unhealthy personal behavior is medically discouraged for individuals, the whole of society legalizes, tolerates, and even encourages the same practices in the population.*

Thomas Schmid and colleagues[54] from the Centers for Disease Control and Prevention summed up the approach discussed here:

> *Health departments that support disincentives for high-fat foods, tax breaks for cafeterias that offer healthy food choices, policies that require zoning ordinances to include sidewalks, or school facilities open to the public might be labeled radical or experimental today; tomorrow, however, they may be considered prudent stewards of the public health.*

In several areas, public health policies are neither new nor experimental. The use of seat belts is a good example of how a law can save lives at minimal cost and with minimal intrusions into individual freedoms. Lead pollution also demonstrates what can be achieved by governmental action. Regulations implemented in the 1970s by the American government forced major reductions or removal of lead from gasoline, paint, water, and consumer products. As a result there was a fourfold reduction in the average blood level of lead of American children over the following 20 years.[55,56]

Barriers against public health policies

A major obstacle to the implementation of public health policies is that industries that profit from unhealthy lifestyles use their considerable resources to resist change. Time and time again we find examples of industries lobbying governments and throwing their money around in order to delay, dilute, or stop laws that threaten their profits. And, more often than not, governments show more sympathy for the financial demands of industry than for the health needs of the general public. Indeed, the political ideology that has gained enormous influence over the past two decades means that governments have been even more business friendly and noninterventionist than ever.

The tobacco industry provides the starkest illustration of this. The US Congress has been very lethargic in passing antismoking legislation. Researchers investigated the likely reason for this and concluded that: "The money that the tobacco industry donates to members of Congress ensures that the tobacco industry will retain its strong influence in the federal tobacco policy process."[57] They showed that in 1991 and 1992 the average senator received $11,600 per year from the tobacco industry. Other researchers studied the California legislature and came to the same conclusion: "Legislative behavior is following tobacco money rather than reflecting constituents' prohealth attitudes on tobacco control."[58]

What is true for the tobacco industry is most certainly true for the agricultural and food industries. Typically, while the health department of governments encourage people to eat less fat, the departments responsible for the agricultural and food industries are far more concerned with appeasing the needs of industry for high sales. Philip James and Ann Ralph[48] of the Rowett Research Institute, Scotland, asserted that: "Analysis of different policies suggest that health issues are readily squeezed out of discussion by economic and vested interests."

An especially informative example of this problem is provided by the way that the meat industry has partially rewritten US dietary guidelines to make them far more industry friendly. In the late 1970s the goal was "eat less meat." This then became "choose lean meat." By 1992 people were encouraged to consume at least two or three servings daily of meat.[59,60]

There is strong evidence that almost everyone has a greatly excessive intake of salt, most of which comes from salt added by manufacturers to processed food. This plays a role in several diseases, especially hypertension and stroke.[61] However, food manufacturers have opposed attempts to reduce the salt content of food. Discussing this question Fiona Goodlee[62], assistant editor of the BMJ, put it as follows:

> . . . *some of the world's major food manufacturers have adopted desperate measures to try to stop governments from recommending salt reduction. Rather than reformulate their products, manufacturers have lobbied governments, refused to co-operate with expert working parties, encouraged misinformation campaigns, and tried to discredit the evidence. . . The tactics over salt are much the same as those used by other sectors of industry. The Sugar Association in the United States and the Sugar Bureau in Britain have waged fierce campaigns against links between sugar and obesity and dental caries.*

National nutrition policies: the case of Norway

In 1976 Norway implemented a pioneering food policy: the Norwegian Nutrition and Food Policy.[63] It recognized that changes in national eating habits require integration of agricultural, economic, and health policy. The policy included consumer and price subsidies, marketing measures, consumer information, and nutrition education in schools. However, this policy clashed with other policies aimed at stimulating agriculture. As is so often the case, economics won the argument; subsidies went to pork, butter, and margarine rather than to potatoes, vegetables, and fruit. Nevertheless, some success was achieved in making the national diet more healthful.[64]

Public health policies and public acceptability

Apart from the resistance of commercial concerns who find their profits threatened, another potential obstacle to the policies advocated here is lack of acceptance by the public. However, the history of seat belt use demonstrates that the public will accept legislation when given evidence to show its importance. A study carried out in the Upper Midwest of the USA revealed considerable support for regulatory controls in the areas of alcohol, tobacco, and, to a lesser extent, high-fat foods, especially with respect to children and youths.[65] It is reasonable to presume that that this degree of acceptance would be at least as great in other countries.

CONCLUSIONS

We now have the knowledge to prevent a substantial fraction of the disease burden that afflicts Western countries. But let us be clear: there is no strong case that prevention will lead to savings in health-care costs. Instead, it is more probable that every dollar saved today on preventing a case of CHD or cancer will translate to at least a dollar spent at a later time for treatment of a chronic, nonfatal disease followed by death from cancer or stroke. In other words, prevention does not save on health-care costs but rather postpones such expenditures. **There is, however, a strong case — indeed an overwhelming case — for prevention, but it is not based on money. Rather, it is based on humanitarian motives: enabling people to add years onto their lives and life onto their years.** Using a blend of **health promotion and government policy, this should be achievable for a small fraction of the dollars spent on high-tech remedial medicine.**

Let us contrast this grand strategy with the one that dominates today's medical orthodoxy. As discussed in preceding chapters, that strategy is focused on the search for new treatments. In other words, it parks an ambulance at the bottom of the cliff rather than building a fence at the top. It follows that curative medicine is always a less attractive option than preventive medicine as avoidable suffering is implicitly accepted. To make matters worse, all too often curative medicine simply does not work. In short, curative medicine has two strikes against it: it does not attempt to prevent preventable diseases and it then achieves an underwhelming level of success in treating them.

This relative lack of success of curative medicine is not due to any lack of research effort. Vast expenditures have been sunk into the quest for new treatments, especially by pharmaceutical companies. The birth of gene therapy – "stillbirth" might prove to be a more accurate term – will expand these expenditures. In stark contrast to this, research in the general area of prevention, including epidemiological research into the causes of disease, intervention trials to test ways to prevent disease, and studies on health promotion, have undoubtedly received far less funding. The conclusion is clear: dollars spent on prevention research achieve far more than do dollars spent on the search for medical treatments, especially those that involve high-tech interventions.

The story of cancer provides compelling support for this view. In 1971 the United States "declared war" on cancer with the passing of the National Cancer Act. Since then no expense has been spared to find a cure. For instance, the estimated 2000 budget of the National Cancer Institute was $3.3 billion. But, as pointed out in chapter nine, there is scant evidence of real progress in terms of five-year survival rates. Yet, during the same 30-year period since 1971, investigations into the relationship between diet and cancer have shown us how one third or more of all cases of cancer can be prevented. There are solid grounds for optimism that within perhaps 20 years this figure will grow to at least 50 percent.

An additional argument in favor of prevention is that in several respects it is environmentally friendly. This is because one component of prevention is a reduction in meat consumption. To produce one pound of beef requires about seven pounds of grain as well as a large input of energy, fertilizers, and water.[66] Meat production also requires far more land usage and is suspected of contributing to global warming because the methane produced by cows is a greenhouse gas. Slashing our consumption of beef is therefore not only an excellent way to improve health but also helps protect the environment.

Health promotion is of much value as a means to prevent such diseases as cancer and CHD. However, that approach has considerable limitations. Far more is likely to be accomplished by public health policies along the lines suggested here. But this will require governments to place national health ahead of narrow commercial interests. This represents a radical reordering of government priorities. But, to be realistic, in today's political climate this is a David versus Goliath battle.

Where do doctors fit into this "new medical order"? Doctors need to recognize their limitations when it comes to therapy. Instead of focusing largely on trying to cure disease, doctors need to act as a pressure group to advocate for change. It is a perfectly realistic goal that broad new coalitions, in which doctors play a prominent role, can successfully pressure for the implementation of public health policies. All that is lacking is the will.

The positions advocated through this book are ones that do not command the support of the powers that be in the world of medical research and medical practice. They would lose money, position, and power to the degree that the reforms would be adopted. This position is not original with us, although we may have assembled the pieces in a more complete fashion than anyone before. Up to now the medical world has been successful in minimizing, disregarding, and simply ignoring this position. We hope that this will change to a significant degree.

References

[1] Clark LC, Combs GF, et al. (1996). Effects of selenium supplementation for cancer prevention in patients with carcinoma of the skin. A randomized trial. *JAMA* 276: 1957-63.

[2] de Lorgeril M, Salen P, et al. (1998). Mediterranean diet pattern in a randomized trial. Prolonged survival and possible reduced cancer rate. *Arch Intern Med* 158: 1181-87.

[3] de Lorgeril M, Salen P, et al. (1999). Mediterranean diet, traditional diet, and the rate of cardiovascular complications after myocardial infarction: final report of the Lyon Heart Study. *Circulation* 99: 779-85.

[4] Stampfer MJ, Hu FB, et al. (2000). Primary prevention of coronary heart disease in women through diet and lifestyle. *N Engl J Med* 343: 16-22.

[5] Flegal KM, Carroll MD, et al. (1998). Overweight and obesity in the United States: prevalence and trends, 1960-1994. *Int J Obesity* 22: 39-47.

[6] Mokdad AH, Serdula MK, et al. (1999). The spread of the obesity epidemic in the United States, 1991-1998. *JAMA* 282: 1519-22.

[7] Siedell JC (1995). Obesity in Europe: scaling an epidemic. *Int J Obesity* 19(Suppl. 3): S1-S4.

[8] Li R, Serdula M, et al. (2000). Trends in fruit and vegetable consumption among adults in 16 US states: behavioral risk factor surveillance system, 1990-1996. *Am J Public Health* 90: 777-81.

[9] Tippett KS, Cleveland LE (1999). In E Frazao. *America's eating habits: changes and consequences.* Washington DC: USDA/ERS, Agricultural Information Bulletin Number 750 (April): 51-70.

[10] Activity and Health Research (1992). *Allied Dunbar National Fitness Survey, a report on activity patterns and fitness levels: main findings.* London: Sports Council and Health Education Authority.

[11] Jones DA, Ainsworth BE, et al. (1998). Moderate leisure-time physical activity: who is meeting the public health recommendations? A national cross-sectional study. *Arch Fam Med* 7: 285-89.

[12] Anon (1998). Self-reported physical inactivity by degree of urbanization – United States, 1996. *MMWR Morb Mortal Wkly Rep* 47: 1097-100.

[13] Farquhar JW, Fortmann SP, et al. (1990). Effects of communitywide education on cardiovascular disease risk factors. The Stanford Five-City Project. *JAMA* 264: 359-65.

[14] Luepker RV, Murray DM, et al. (1994). Community education for cardiovascular disease prevention: risk factor changes in the Minnesota Heart Health Program. *Am J Public Health* 84: 1383-93.

[15] Carleton RA, Lasater TM, et al. (1995). The Pawtucket Heart Health Program: community changes in cardiovascular risk factors and projected disease risk. *Am J Public Health* 85: 777-85.

[16] Winkleby MA, Feldman HA, Murray DM (1997). Joint analysis of three U.S. community intervention trials for reduction of cardiovascular risk. *J Clin Epidemiol* 50: 645-58.

[17] Goodman RM, Wheeler FC, Lee PR (1995). Evaluation of the Heart To Heart Project: lessons from a community-based chronic disease prevention project. *Am J Health Promot* 9: 443-55.

[18] Brownson RC, Smith CA, et al. (1996). Preventing cardiovascular disease through community-based risk reduction: the Bootheel Heart Health Project. *Am J Public Health* 86: 206-13.

[19] Puska P, Nissinen A, et al. (1985). The community based strategy to prevent coronary heart disease: conclusions from the ten years of North Karelia project. *Ann Rev Public Health* 6: 147-93.

[20] Valkonen T (1992). Trends in regional and socio-economic mortality differentials in Finland. *Int J Health Sci* 3: 157-66.

[21] Hoffmeister H, Mensink GB, et al. (1996). Reduction of coronary heart disease risk factors in the German Cardiovascular Prevention study. *Prev Med* 25: 135-45.

[22] Baxter T, Milner P, et al. (1997). A cost effective, community based heart health promotion project in England: prospective comparative study. *BMJ* 315: 582-85.

[23] Reger B, Wootan MG, Booth-Butterfield S (1999). Using mass media to promote healthy eating: a community–based demonstration project. *Prev Med* 29: 414-21.

[24] Dixon H, Boland R, et al. (1998). Public reaction to Victoria's "2 Fruit 'n' 5 Veg Day" campaign and reported consumption of fruit and vegetables. *Prev Med* 27: 572-82.

[25] Sorensen G, Morris DM, et al. (1992). Work-site nutrition intervention and employees' dietary habits: the Treatwell program. *Am J Public Health* 82: 877-80.

[26] Sorensen G, Stoddard A, et al. (1999). Increasing fruit and vegetable consumption through worksites and families in the Treatwell 5-a-Day Study. *Am J Public Health* 89: 54-60.

[27] Jeffery RW, Forster JL, et al. (1993). The Healthy Worker Project: a work-site intervention for weight control and smoking cessation. *Am J Public Health* 83: 395-401.

[28] Imperial Cancer Research Fund OXCHECK Study Group (1994). Effectiveness of health checks conducted by nurses in primary care: results of the OXCHECK study after one year. *BMJ* 308: 308-12.

[29] Imperial Cancer Research Fund OXCHECK Study Group (1995). Effectiveness of health checks conducted by nurses in primary care: final results of the OXCHECK study. *BMJ* 310: 1099-104.

[30] Family Heart Study Group (1994). Randomised controlled trial evaluating cardiovascular screening and intervention in general practice: principal results of British Family Heart Study. *BMJ* 308: 313-20.

[31] Brunner E, White I, et al. (1997). Can dietary interventions change diet and cardiovascular risk factors? A meta-analysis of randomized controlled trials. *Am J Public Health* 87: 1415-22.

[32] Field K, Thorogood M, et al. (1995). Strategies for reducing coronary risk factors in primary care: which is most cost effective? *BMJ* 310: 1109-12.

[33] Lindholm LH, Ekbom T, et al. (1995). The impact of health care advice given in primary care on cardiovascular risk. *BMJ* 310: 1105-09.

[34] Rose G (1992). *The strategy of preventive medicine.* Oxford: Oxford University Press.

[35] Meier KJ, Licari MJ (1997). The effect of cigarette taxes on cigarette consumption, 1955 through 1994. *Am J Public Health* 87: 1126-30.

[36] Townsend J (1996). Price and consumption of tobacco. *Br Med Bull* 52: 132-42.

[37] Townsend J, Roderick P, Cooper J (1994). Cigarette smoking by socioeconomic group, sex, and age: effects of price income, and health publicity. *BMJ* 309: 923-27.

[38] Stephens T, Pedersen LL, et al. (1997). The relationship of cigarette prices and no-smoking bylaws to the prevalence of smoking in Canada. *Am J Public Health* 87: 1519-21.

[39] Anderson P, Lehto G (1994). Prevention policies. *Br Med Bull* 50: 171-85.

[40] World Health Organization Regional Office for Europe (1988). *The Adelaide recommendations: healthy public policy.* Geneva: World Health Organization.

[41] French SA, Jeffery RW, et al. (1997). A pricing strategy to promote low-fat snack choices through vending machines. *Am J Public Health* 87: 849-51.

[42] Jeffery RW, French SA, et al. (1994). An environmental intervention to increase fruit and salad purchases in a cafeteria. *Prev Med* 23: 788-92.

[43] French SA, Story M, et al. (1997). Pricing strategy to promote fruit and vegetable purchase in high school cafeterias. *J Am Diet Assoc* 97: 1008-10.

[44] Nestle M, Wing R, et al. (1998). Behavioral and social influence on food choice. *Nutr Rev* 56: S50-S64.

[45] Advertising Age (1999). *100 leading national advertisers: 44th annual report.* (September 27): S1-S46.

[46] Kotz K, Story M (1994). Food advertisements during children's Saturday morning television programming: Are they consistent with dietary recommendations? J Am Diet Assoc 94: 1296-300.

[47] Ostbye T, Pomerleau, et al. (1993). Food and nutrition in Canadian "prime time" television commercials. *Can J Public Health* 84: 370-74.

[48] James WPT, Ralph A (1992). National strategies for dietary change. In M Marmot, Elliott P, eds. *Coronary heart disease. From aetiology to public health.* Oxford: Oxford University Press: 525-40.

[49] James WPT (1995). A public health approach to the problem of obesity. *Int J Obesity* 19(Suppl. 3): S37-S45.

[50] Nestle M (1998). Toward more healthful dietary patterns – A matter of policy. *Public Health Rep* 113: 420-23.

[51] Jeffery RW (1991). Population perspectives on the prevention and treatment of obesity in minority populations. *Am J Clin Nutr* 53: 1621S-24S.

[52] Nestle M, Jacobson MF (2000). Halting the obesity epidemic: a public health policy approach. *Public Health Rep* 115: 12-24.

[53] Blackburn H (1992). Community programmes in coronary heart disease prevention health promotion: changing community behavior. In: Marmot M, Elliott P, eds. *Coronary heart disease. From aetiology to public health.* Oxford: Oxford University Press: 495-514.

[54] Schmid TL, Pratt M, Howze E (1995). Policy as intervention: environmental and policy approaches to the prevention of cardiovascular disease. *Am J Public Health* 85: 1207-11.

[55] Pirkle JL, Brody DJ, et al. (1994). The decline in blood lead levels in the United States. *JAMA* 272: 284-91.

[56] Brody DJ, Pirkle JL, et al. (1994). Blood lead levels in the US population. *JAMA* 272: 277-83.

[57] Moore S, Wolfe SM, et al. (1994). Epidemiology of failed tobacco control legislation. *JAMA* 272: 1171-75.

[58] Glantz SA, Begay ME (1994). Tobacco industry campaign contributions are affecting tobacco control policymaking in California. *JAMA* 272: 1176-82.

[59] Nestle M (1993). Food lobbies, the food pyramid and U.S. nutrition policy. *Int J Health Serv* 23: 483-96.

[60] Nestle M (1994). The politics of dietary guidance - A new opportunity. *Am J Public Health* 84: 713-15.

[61] Kaplan NM (2000). Evidence in favor of moderate dietary sodium reduction. *Am J Hypertension* 13: 8-13.

[62] Goodlee F (1996). The food industry fights for salt. *BMJ* 312: 1239-40.

[63] Klepp K, Forster JL (1985). The Norwegian Nutrition and Food Policy: an integrated approach to a public health problem. *J Public Health Policy* 6: 447-63.

[64] Norum KR, Johansson L, et al. (1997). Nutrition and food policy in Norway: effects on reduction of coronary heart disease. *Nutr Rev* 55: S32-S39.

[65] Jeffery RW, Forster JL, et al. (1990). Community attitudes toward public policies to control alcohol, tobacco, and high-fat food consumption. *Am J Prev Med* 6: 12-19.

[66] Whitney EN, Rolfes SR (1999). *Understanding nutrition.* Belmont, CA: Wadsworth Publishing Company.

Postscript

Norman J. Temple, Andrew Thompson

"The reasonable man adapts himself to the world: the unreasonable man persists in trying to adapt the world to himself. Therefore all progress depends on the unreasonable man." George Bernard Shaw in *Reason*

At the heart of large organizations or movements there is usually a core mythology. Armies, political movements, and religions rely on the core mythology to motivate their members. Hand-in-hand with the core mythology, members are pressured to stay "in line." To do so means rewards of various sorts: praise, career advancement, and perhaps money. But to question the core mythology risks serious negative consequences.

We see much the same pattern in medicine. At medical school, future physicians are imbued with a faith in high-tech treatments. The core mythology, which is implicitly written into the medical curriculum, can be summarized as: high-tech treatment and the latest drugs are the best treatment, they should be used often (unless there is clear evidence to the contrary), and cost of treatment is not a relevant issue. Doctors who embrace the core mythology and act on it in their daily practice are much more likely to ride the gravy train, while those who act independently can expect a lack of career advancement and perhaps even censure by their colleagues. After all, since medicating with statins, the use of right heart catheters, and screening for prostate cancer are all the accepted wisdom, it follows that any physician who is unenthusiastic in their use must be guilty of misconduct.

The following is perhaps the ultimate example of this mind-set? One of us (Norman Temple) recently visited an operating theatre in Cape Town that holds a special place in the history of medicine. For it was there that in the late 1960s a series of heart transplants was carried out that mesmerized the

189

A. Thompson and N.J. Temple (eds.), Ethics, Medical Research, and Medicine, 189–192.
© 2001 Kluwer Academic Publishers. Printed in the Netherlands.

world. Surely this was the future of medicine: technological advances to bring people back from certain death and give them a new lease on life. However, it seems that this procedure is not quite the miracle of modern medicine that many believe it to be. While writing this Postscript a report was published giving the findings of a German study.[1] Contrary to the widely accepted "truth" most people given heart transplants had a no better survival than those left on the waiting list due to a lack of donors. The only patients who appear to benefit are those facing imminent death.

The boast is often heard that "America has the best medical system in the world." The hollowness of this statement was exposed by an analysis published in *JAMA*.[2] The researcher estimated that 225,000 people die in the USA each year from iatrogenic causes, mostly from nosocomial infections (infections contracted in hospitals) and from nonerror adverse effects of medications. Incredible as it may seem, this makes iatrogenic causes the third leading cause of death in the USA, well ahead of cerebrovascular disease. This finding should rate a 9.6 on the Richter Scale. While this problem clearly goes well beyond high-tech medicine, it speaks volumes as to the incredible overconfidence that pervades all aspects of the American medical system. This must inevitably extend into high-tech areas.

What we see, time and time again, are new high-tech medical "advances" which are accepted based on what is later found to be weak evidence. They almost invariably come with a high price tag. As a result medicine becomes evermore expensive. But the general population, who, in every respect, have to pay the price, are not receiving the medical care that they need. Of course, many medical advances are successful; no one denies that. But the medical establishment has a rather poor track record of sorting the real advances from the false promises.

Those who are in the business of selling products for use by physicians understand all this. Indeed, their marketing strategy is based on it. What we see is a synergistic relationship: commercial interests, especially the pharmaceutical industry, push new products, using all manner of misleading information to exaggerate the goods on offer, while the medical profession has a mind-set that leaves it highly receptive to promises of new "advances."

Perhaps the group best able to clean up this mess are academic researchers. Only they are in a position to act independently and objectively evaluate medical treatments. Unfortunately, large numbers of academic researchers have had limitations placed on their independence. One reason for this is that many receive funding from pharmaceutical companies. Often researchers may suffer from the same self-imposed restrictions that affect so many physicians: to question medical "advances" may be somehow out of bounds, "thought crime" in Orwellian English.

The mind-set that prevails in medicine is also seen in many other spheres of human endeavor. All over the world the marriage of commercialization and high-tech advances have proven a mixed blessing. Consider these examples:

- The mass production of cars and gasoline has been a major factor in such problems as urban sprawl, widespread air pollution, and global warming.
- Nuclear energy has created huge amounts of highly toxic waste which will remain a hazard for thousands of years.
- Vast numbers of toxic chemicals are invented, manufactured, and used widely but only decades later are their dangers identified.
- Highly processed food is a major cause of the epidemic of chronic diseases that plagues all Western societies.
- TV: this speaks for itself.

In each case commercial interests have used their powers – especially by advertising and by pressuring governments – to force widespread acceptance of these "advances." Anyone questioning their benefits was seen as antiprogress. But, in each case it was slowly realized that "progress" can have a dark side.

The authors of this book are most certainly not antiprogress. They both take planes, as indeed one did from Switzerland to visit the other in Canada. They both drive cars in places with inadequate public transport. If ethics means anything, it means taking a balanced view of a complex situation that has conflicting interests. That certainly applies to the above examples. And it most certainly applies to medical ethics.

In the introduction to this book we briefly discussed contrasting world views. Let us revisit that question. In general, the problems created by commercialization and high-tech solutions to human needs (real or imagined) can also be seen, in part, as contempt for nature and the environment. We see this clearly in the development of nuclear energy, toxic chemicals, and highly processed food. Clearly, with nuclear energy and toxic chemicals we are despoiling the environment while with highly processed food we are forgetting that they are so unnatural that disease is the almost inevitable consequence.

So also with medicine. At the heart of so many attempts to fix health problems is a belief that nature can and should be mastered. This arrogant attitude has met with far more failures than successes. A more rational approach is the opposite. We should respect nature and endeavor to live in harmony with it. That includes recognizing and accepting that we are creatures of the natural world. Health comes from following that principle: a natural diet (comparable to that eaten by our paleolithic ancestors), exercise, and not smoking. Such a formula may be less intellectually appealing than the quest for genetic therapies but it will undoubtedly be of far more benefit to humanity. The world will be better for it.

References

[1] Deng MC, De Meester JMJ, et al. (2000). Effect of receiving a heart transplant: analysis of a national cohort entered on to a waiting list, stratified by heart failure severity. *BMJ* 321: 540-05.

[2] Starfield B (2000). Is US health really the best in the world? *JAMA* 283: 483-85.

Index